The
Lyme-Autism
Connection

The
Lyme-Autism
Connection

Unveiling the Shocking Link Between Lyme Disease and Childhood Developmental Disorders

An Investigative Report

By **Bryan Rosner**
With **Tami Duncan**

Foreword by
Robert Bransfield, M.D., D.F.A.P.A

BioMed Publishing Group

BioMed Publishing Group
P.O. Box 9012
South Lake Tahoe, CA 96158
www.LymeBook.com

**For related books and DVDs visit us online at <u>www.lymebook.com</u>.
Visit the LIA Foundation online at <u>www.liafoundation.org</u>.**

Disclaimer

Acknowledgements

Tami's Acknowledgements

Thank you to Troy, Jenna and Michael for allowing me to go forth on this mission. This book is dedicated to all of the Michael's and Jenna's and Ryan's and Alex's and Aiden's and the children we don't know but fight for everyday to find answers to help them in their healing journey. I'd also like to acknowledge the moms and dads who are with us on this mission, but too sick to help; you are in our prayers.

Bryan's Acknowledgements

I would like to thank all of the researchers, parents, and physicians who have been looking into this connection for years. I was only able to write this book by standing on their shoulders. There are far too many of these people to list by name. I would also like to thank Tami Duncan and the LIA Foundation for providing me with the opportunity to be part of such an important and fascinating area of research. Finally, I must thank my wife and new son for supporting me during the process of writing this book.

I would also like to thank those who reviewed this book prior to publication: Connie Strasheim, James Schaller, M.D., Scott Forsgren, Drew Kondo, and Nancy Ng.

Statements from Scientists, Researchers and Physicians

"When a pregnant woman is infected with Lyme disease, not only is she subject to its devastation, but her baby is, too."

—John Drulle, MD
Urgent care and private practice physician

"Accumulation of experimental evidence also points to potential for peri-, pre- and postnatal infections as causes for several neurodevelopmental disorders such as schizophrenia, autism, cerebral palsy and mental retardation."

—Excerpt from the book "Neuropsychiatric Disorders and Infection," edited by Hossein Fatemi, MD, Ph.D., Associate Professor, University of Minnesota Medical Center

"An association between Lyme disease and other tick-borne infections during fetal development and in infancy with autism, autism spectrum disorders (ASD) and autistic symptoms has been noted by numerous clinicians and parents."

—Medical Hypothesis journal article written by Robert C. Bransfield, MD, Jeffrey S. Wulfman, MD, William T. Harvey, MD, Anju I. Usman, MD

"An observant parent's evidence may be disproved but should never be ignored."

—Lancet, 1951

"Lyme produces a micro-edema, or swelling in the brain. This affects your ability to process information. It's like finding out that there's LSD in the punch, and you're not sure what's going to happen next or if you're going to be in control of your own thoughts."

—Bernard Raxlen, MD

"Great diversity of clinical expression of signs and symptoms of gestational Lyme borreliosis parallels the diversity of prenatal Syphilis. It is documented that transplacental transmission of the spirochete from mother to fetus is possible...Autopsy and clinical studies have associated gestational Lyme borreliosis with various medical problems including fetal death, hydrocephalus, cardiovascular anomalies, neonatal respiratory distress, hyperbilirubinemia, intrauterine growth retardation, cortical blindness, sudden infant death syndrome, and maternal toxemia of pregnancy."

—AB MacDonald, MD, Souhampton Hospital, New York, abstract taken from a study published in 1989.

"Relapsing-fever borreliosis caused by Borrelia duttonii [a strain of Lyme bacteria] is a common cause of complications of pregnancy, miscarriage, and neonatal death in sub-Saharan Africa...B. duttonii infection during pregnancy results in intrauterine growth retardation, as well as placental damage and inflammation, impaired fetal circulation, and decreased maternal hemoglobin levels...Spirochetes frequently cross the maternal-fetal barrier, resulting in congenital infection."

— Christer Larsson, et al., Department of Molecular Biology Umea University, Sweden.

Lyme-Autism Resources

Lyme-Induced Autism (LIA) Foundation

www.liafoundation.org

Lyme-Induced Autism (LIA) Foundation
Conference DVD Sets

www.lymebook.com/autism

Table of Contents

Foreword by Robert Bransfield, MD

What causes autism? If this question could be easily answered we would know by now. Although some cases can be clearly explained, most cannot. Most often, it appears to be caused by a genetic predisposition interacting with environmental triggers. What are the genes that predispose to autism? What are the environmental triggers? What exactly is the pathological process that results in autism? How can we explain the range of different symptoms associated with autism spectrum disorder? Why is the incidence of autism spectrum disorder increasing? What can we do to prevent and treat this condition? These are the basic questions we need to keep asking until they are fully answered. Every possible cause, every possible contributing factor and every possible explanation must be explored thoroughly until these puzzles are solved.

Theoretical biology looks at chronic low grade infections as the cause of many diseases. From general medical research there is a growing body of evidence that infections and immune reactions to these infections contribute to numerous health disorders. Rubella and Syphilis have been known to cause autism, but research has demonstrated an ever growing list of other infections also associated with autism that now includes Herpes simplex, Herpes-6, Mycoplasma, Borna virus, Chlamydia, Malaria, Cytomegalovirus, Varicella, Toxoplasmosis, Lyme disease, other tick-borne diseases and yet unrecognized infections. At the same time that this evidence has been accumulating in the scientific literature, many parents, physicians and other clinicians have noticed an association between Lyme and other tick-borne diseases and autism spectrum disorder. The LIA Foundation (a description of which can be found in a few pages) was created to better coordinate efforts to explore this association and it has resulted in better communication and accelerated progress. The weight of evidence associating tick-borne diseases with autism spectrum disorders keeps increasing and further attention to and exploration of this connection is needed until answers are indisputable.

This book will look at some pieces of the puzzle, in particular the Lyme/tick-borne disease association with autism spectrum disorder. This is the first book devoted to the subject. It will not be the last. I hope you find it interesting, educational and thought-provoking. As long as children are afflicted with this condition, we can never be complacent and accept the status quo. We need constant effort until this disease has been fully understood and eradicated.

Robert C. Bransfield, MD, DFAPA
Red Bank, New Jersey

Information for the Reader

THE LIA FOUNDATION

The LIA Foundation (Lyme-Induced Autism Foundation) is the most important resource that will be mentioned in this book. The LIA Foundation is the hub for current Lyme-autism research. It brings together parents, patients, and practitioners from around the globe.

This book is intended as a high-level overview of the Lyme-autism connection. The LIA Foundation can provide more in-depth, updated information. Autism medicine is evolving rapidly, and the LIA Foundation is the place to stay connected with the latest news, treatment announcements, and research.

As you will read in the next section, because information and research are evolving so quickly, this book does not include detailed treatment guidelines. The LIA Foundation will do their best to be your source for updated treatment guidelines as new information becomes available.

The LIA Foundation was established in 2005 by several mothers of children affected by childhood developmental disorders, including Tami Duncan, co-author of this book. According to the foundation website, www.liafoundation.org, their mission is the following:

1. To educate, through our awareness programs, parents, physicians and the community, about the importance of testing for Borrelia, mycoplasma and many other infections in children with Autism Spectrum Disorder.

2. To educate the autism community, both doctors and parents, about how to find a doctor knowledgeable in Borrelia,

mycoplasma and multiple infections and connect parents with mentors who can help guide them through their journey.

3. To assist in coordinating future medical studies to help with treatments, information and education.

The LIA Foundation conducts a radio show aired approximately once a month. The show is called "The Lyme-Autism Connection." You can learn more about the show at www.autismone.org. The foundation sponsors and participates in numerous conferences, and they submit articles to various Lyme- and Autism-related publications, including the *Townsend Letter for Doctors and Patients* (www.townsendletter.com) and *Public Health Alert* (www.publichealthalert.org).

The foundation has an advisory board which, at the time of this writing, is comprised of the following specialists:

> **Robert C. Bransfield, MD, DFAPA, PC**
> **Lee Cowden, MD FACC, MD(H)**
> **Dietrich Klinghardt, MD, PhD**
> **Warren Levin, MD PLLC, FACN, FAAEM, FAAFP (ret)**
> **Janelle Love, MD**
> **Ian R. Luepker, ND, DHANP**
> **Anju Usman, MD**
> **Toby Watkinson, DC**
> **Jeff Wulfman, MD**
> **Therese H. Yang, MD, FAAFP**
> **Amy Derksen, ND**
> **James Schaller, MD, MAR, DABPN**

The LIA Foundation plays a critical role in the advancement of research on the Lyme-autism connection. Modern medicine tends to over-categorize, separate, and compartmentalize diseases. Hence, there are plenty of doctors, researchers, and scientists studying autism, and there are plenty studying Lyme disease. But there are very few studying the *connection* between Lyme disease and autism—this is the role played by the LIA Foundation.

The LIA Foundation website (www.liafoundation.org) is a wealth of information, and you should visit the website before taking any other action. If you are a parent, caretaker, family member, or friend of a person with a developmental disorder, the LIA Foundation is an excellent resource. The Foundation can help connect you with a physician in your area proficient in the treatment of both Lyme disease and autism.

INTRODUCTION TO THIS BOOK

You should be aware of the following information, which clarifies what this book offers and what it does not:

1. Parents must absolutely not take drastic actions in response to this book. The Lyme-autism connection is not yet sufficiently substantiated to warrant big changes in how autistic children are treated and managed. In the event that you do feel warranted in changing your child's treatment program, do so only under the close supervision of a licensed, trusted physician who is proficient in treating Lyme disease and/or autism (see Chapter 7 for more information on finding a physician).

2. This book is not the final word, but instead, a first question. The area of Lyme-autism research is rapidly developing. This book presents data which is current through the time period in which the book was researched and written. To stay up-to-date, remain connected with the LIA Foundation.

3. This book was written specifically to elucidate the scientific evidence substantiating the Lyme-autism connection. The book *was not* written to provide a basic education in Lyme disease

or in autism. If you are unfamiliar with these two diseases, you will need to seek education elsewhere. Appendix B has been provided to introduce you to some of the key elements of current Lyme disease treatment, politics, controversy, and associated concepts. Appendix B is an excerpt from *The Top 10 Lyme Disease Treatments*, available from www.LymeBook.com.

4. Before reading this book, you should know that complexity and controversy are hallmarks of both Lyme disease and autism.

5. Because the Lyme-autism connection is an emerging area of medicine, not yet well-defined or well-studied, there are not many published research papers on the topic. There are thousands of available studies on autism, and thousands of available studies on Lyme disease, but only a few that look at the connection between the afflictions. Therefore, instead of reviewing studies that connect Lyme disease and autism, this book will focus primarily on independent Lyme disease studies and independent autism studies, and attempt to make meaningful comparisons between the studies in an effort to extrapolate fundamental information about the Lyme-autism connection.

Although not many in number, there are a few studies that do examine the direct connection between Lyme disease and autism. Obviously, these studies are of key importance. They were given special attention during the research phase of writing this book.

6. There are two areas of interest that people learning about the Lyme-autism connection will inevitably encounter: First, the connection between autism and Lyme disease specifically, and second, the connection between autism and infections in general. Science suggests that, while Lyme disease may be one of the infections involved in autism, numerous other infections are also involved.

This book focuses primarily on the connection between autism and Lyme disease specifically, not the connection between autism and infections in general.

The reason this book focuses on Lyme disease instead of infections in general is twofold. First, there is already a tremendous amount of information available focusing on infections in general and their relationship to autism, while there is a limited amount of information focusing specifically on the relationship between Lyme disease and autism.

Second, unlike many other infections, the number of Lyme disease cases in the United States and abroad is skyrocketing. Accordingly, a specific focus on Lyme disease is warranted as Lyme disease has reached epidemic proportions.

7. This book approaches the topic of the Lyme-autism connection with a heavier focus on the Lyme disease component, not the autism component.

8. We are not offering specific treatment guidelines for the Lyme-autism connection because so little is known about the disease. It is certainly true that many physicians are successfully dealing with the Lyme-autism connection. However, their approaches are almost always highly customized to the patient at hand and also very fluid and adaptable as new information becomes available. Both of these qualities of a treatment program (customization and rapid adaptation) are completely incompatible with static, printed books.

Thus, treating patients with both Lyme disease and autism is highly complex and beyond the scope of this book. We suggest reading everything you can on the topics of Lyme disease and autism, and staying connected to the LIA Foundation, which will be the primary source for updated information as the weeks, months, and years pass. Since no child is the clone of another, and since no two children will be treated in the same way, the single most important thing you can do is to find a physician who is literate in treating the diseases. Instructions for finding such a physician are provided in Chapter 7.

An additional proactive step you can take in staying up-to-date on current treatment theory is to attend the LIA Foundation conferences, if possible. If you cannot attend the conferences, you can also view them live on a webcast made available by ZenWorks Productions, www.zenworksproductions.com. The webcast is live so you will need to tune in during the conferences. You can find out when the upcoming conferences are taking place and get additional information at the ZenWorks website (above) or the LIA Foundation website (www.liafoundation.org).

Alternatively, you can also acquire the DVD recordings from recent LIA Foundation conferences. Purchase these DVDs from www.lymebook.com/autism. These DVDs are tremendously important; they allow you to see and hear first-hand the researchers and clinicians on the front lines of this emerging field of research, and the included presentations offer differing and broad perspectives on the Lyme-autism connection. Presenters have included Charles Ray Jones, M.D., Robert Bransfield, M.D., Warren Levin, M.D., Richard Horowitz, M.D., Richie Shoemaker, M.D., among others. In addition to sharing the science of the Lyme-autism connection, these physicians also share the treatments and approaches which they have found most helpful in their practices for dealing with Lyme disease and autism.

Preface: Getting Personal With Bryan and Tami

Before diving into the science of the Lyme-autism connection, we felt you would appreciate knowing where the authors are coming from on a personal level. After all, as human beings who feel, experience, think and live, our life stories influence everything we do—including writing books. This book was written by Bryan Rosner with contribution from Tami Duncan, and below, you can read about our personal experiences with Lyme disease and autism, and find out how those experiences have shaped our lives and directed the projects with which we have become involved.

TAMI'S PREFACE: RESEARCH AND QUESTIONS BRING NEW HOPE

It seems like yesterday when my beautiful baby boy was born. He was born right on time; on his due date, in fact. He was healthy and had a great APGAR score. He seemed happy to be in my inexperienced arms; I had never even held a baby before.

As he began to grow and develop, there were many times that I thought this boy must be some kind of genius. I swear I heard him say "Elmo" at just six months of age. He was my perfect little boy. The lady at work said she had never seen such great, fine motor skills, as he could take apart mechanical things that had just the tiniest of screws.

I had the usual arsenal of baby books to track his progress. He made most of the milestones on the check-off list. The things he hadn't accomplished, the doctor said it was "because he was a boy and they can just take longer." Okay...well, I didn't know any better. He was my first-born; who was I to question the decades of experience that the grandmas and doctors have?

When it came time for preschool, my guy seemed to cling to me much more than the other kids. I remember crying outside the preschool door, because I could still hear him crying for me. They assured me that he would calm down after just a few minutes in the classroom. I knew this was right in my head, but my heart told me that it wasn't. The teachers also raved about how smart he was; he could stack blocks much higher than the other kids. A sense of self-satisfaction filled me. I'm doing well.

When he was four and in pre-kindergarten, I noticed that he wasn't doing the same things as the other children. His speech seemed more slurred; his coloring was more scribbly. He was also notorious for playing alone on the playground or looking for bugs by himself. My poor baby, just like his mommy, had a hard time connecting with other kids. I asked the preschool teacher if she thought there was any problem. She said, "Oh no, don't worry about it. Sometimes the boys just take longer." Hmmm.

Kindergarten came and more differences began appearing between him and the other children. My son couldn't jump, run fast, hop, read, or write his name. All of the other kids could do this. I finally realized that I couldn't listen to what other people were saying and had to go with my "mommy gut." I made a list of the things my son couldn't do. This list took up two pages. I presented this to his teacher, and she said I was right. But in private school, they really don't know what to do. I'll always be grateful for Mrs. Smith who spent time praying about my son, and what to do next. She finally came to me with the answer.

As she was perusing through the educational supply store one day, a lady asked Mrs. Smith what she was looking for. She told her all about my son. This lady just happened to be a special education teacher. She asked Mrs. Smith about his symptoms and determined that he needed an evaluation for sensory integration disorder. When Mrs. Smith told me this, I remember having to write it down... "Sensory integration disorder. What is this?" I'd never heard of it. But by researching online, it sounded right.

Finally, we got an evaluation for SID and speech. I remember my heart falling to my feet when I saw Miss Beth evaluate him. He could do much less than even I had thought. We walked away with a plan to start occupational therapy and speech therapy twice a week.

I thought we were all set; that we had our answer. But then in first grade, the gap between his skills and other children's widened even further. He was not reading well. He couldn't keep up in any subject except science. When I asked our school district for help, they told me they couldn't help him until he was three years behind the other kids. This was a lie. This lie enraged me enough to start telling everyone about it. By just a fluke, I told a total stranger in the cell phone store this story. His sister-in-law happened to be an advocate for children with special needs. This began our journey into the world of autism.

After much bureaucratic baloney, I took my son to one of the leading pediatric neurologists in Southern California. We walked out with an autism diagnosis. Was this devastating? It was bittersweet. I wasn't destroyed, because I looked at this as an opportunity to finally have some things to work on. Autism opens up the doors for many other therapies and resources. When a kid just has sensory integration disorder, it appears that the only thing to do is occupational therapy.

My son was seven years old when we got the diagnosis of autism spectrum disorder. It took me about one year to find information on biomedical treatments for him. At that point, he was eight years old. His age was past the "window of opportunity," as many people call it. No chance for early intervention here. The mommy guilt set in "...I should have, would have, could have, if I had known...."

We began treatment with a DAN (Defeat Autism Now) doctor. Immediately, we began the gluten-free/casein-free diet. We tested and treated other issues such as metal toxicity, yeast overgrowth, viral issues, and vitamin/mineral deficiencies. At this time, my little guy flourished. He began reading and jumped from a kindergarten to 3rd grade reading level in just three months. His tantrums, compliance, and behavioral issues diminished drastically. The progress we saw was amazing. He still had autism but was improving significantly.

During this time, I started noticing that I was very tired, irritable, and seemed to get sick a lot. I was getting ear and sinus infections, and frequently having weird hallucinogenic dreams. I went to the doctor many times and was always hurried out with yet another antibiotic.

It wasn't until November, 2005 that I received my wake up call. I woke up one Sunday morning with no voice. No sound louder than a whisper would come out. I had no other symptoms. I wasn't sick, just no voice. I went to the doctor and was given another round of antibiotics. After a week with no improvements, I went to an ear, nose, and throat specialist. He noted that one of my vocal cords looked paralyzed. He thought it was probably a virus and that my voice should come back soon. He said if it didn't come back in a month, to call and make an appointment. A month! I thought to myself, "Are you kidding me?"

After four weeks without a voice, I contacted my son's DAN doctor and he referred me to a Naturopath in his office. Luckily she squeezed me in quickly, because at this point, I had no patience left. She took a history, and talked about testing. She read off a list of tests she wanted to do. I handed over the credit card and said, "Run them." I wanted my voice back before Christmas.

A few weeks later, the office faxed the lab results over to me. My voice had magically come back after two months, but I still wanted answers. I was shocked, to say the least, when my labs showed multiple infections. In fact, the test that was the most staggering was this Western Blot she ran. It showed that I was 100% positive for Lyme disease. I didn't even know what this was and had to Google it. I was blown away to find that it is caused by a tick. I still attest that under no circumstances do I camp; I hotel! I never remember a tick bite of any sort whatsoever. But yet, here it was. I had Lyme disease, and the symptoms of it to boot.

I told my son's doctor about my diagnosis. He said to me, "You know, some of these autistic kids are testing positive for Lyme, too." What? What did he just say? But how? I went home and Googled that too and found an entire group of moms online on a Yahoo! group called Lyme-Autism; hundreds of them in fact, in which the mom was sick with Lyme and the child had autism and Lyme disease. I called the DAN doctor and said I wanted our whole family tested.

Luckily my daughter and husband were spared. But my little boy, at this time nine years old, still having autism, was positive for Lyme. In a twisted way, I was happy. Finally we had another piece of his "autism puzzle." You see, we had hit a wall or plateau with his current treatments. We had done almost everything and weren't able to pull out any more improvements. This Lyme disease diagnosis provided a scary, yet realistic reality that we did have things to work at. If we treated the Lyme infection, we might be able to pull out more improvements.

I told one of the other autism mommies about my son having Lyme and she said, "Oh, so you gave it to him." I just walked away, stunned and devastated. Was she right? Well, if she was, I would have never given him anything on purpose. Squash the guilt; it's all I can do. I can't help but feel guilty, but I know that it's unproductive, ridiculous, and just plain old stupid. I learned that we pass on lots of our immunity and antibodies to our children. It's a natural process of child-birth.

So there we went, mommy and son on a similar journey together. We are fighting to be well, fighting for our health. I was able to get a new understanding of some of the things my son would go through. My Lyme disease presented itself mostly neurologically. I was having word-finding problems, some slurred speech, a lot of forgetfulness, lack of focus, light and sound sensitivity—just to name a few. I was put on a diet free of gluten and casein. Now I realize just how difficult it must be for our kids to go on this diet. But I also realize how necessary it is. I felt the "leaky gut" syndrome and pain involved when I would cheat on this diet.

We both were under the care of an LLMD (Lyme-literate medical doctor). I seemed to be getting sicker and my son's liver couldn't tolerate the medication. I was told that he would need to go on IV antibiotics once his yeast was under control. The last statement is laughable. You see, we had never been able to get his yeast under control. So now what could we do? No Lyme treatment? How could we recover if we could not get rid of this horrible bug?

I dug up the number of a woman named Kathy. Kathy is considered the expert mom on Lyme disease on the Internet. I called her, pissed off. We talked about how the Lyme doctors don't understand autism and how the majority of autism doctors have no clue how to treat or even test for Lyme. Where does this leave our kids? In addition, I had read online that Dr. Dietrich Klinghardt was testing autistic children and found that many of them had Lyme. Was this bigger than we thought? Was it more than just these few hundred kids? Could it be thousands? This conversation with Kathy was pivotal.

We talked about holding a "think tank" and bringing these doctors together to come up with some answers for our kids. But would doctors fly across the country at the request of two desperate moms? No, they wouldn't. We decided that we needed to form a foundation; a non-profit, to have some validity behind us. Within just one month we were set up, making contact with doctors, and planning our first event.

We filed papers for our non-profit we refer to as the LIA Foundation at the end of September 2006, and had our think tank just three months later in January 2007. The doctors came—the passionate doctors, that is. We had no money to bring them in, or even to pay for their hotel room. We had only enough to get the meeting space, some coffee, and a light breakfast. I'm forever grateful for these doctors who came and spent the weekend passionately discussing these kids and what they could do to bring about healing.

A blessing for us personally came out of this think tank. A mom, Carmen, had called me and begged me to invite her daughter's doctor to the think tank. She said that he was able to get her daughter, who was bedridden, out with her friends and off all medications. "Okay," I said, "I'll call and talk to him." I called Toby's office and he personally answered the phone. We talked for 30 minutes and he told me about his methods—which were, indeed, outside the box. But, I figured, who was I to judge? If he's healing kids and adults, let's check it out.

My son's DAN doctor was at the think tank and said, "I want you to take Michael to see Toby Watkinson." After seeing his presentation, I was in total agreement. Dr. Watkinson has been able to pull my son out of his plateau and show a new level of healing and improvements. We are on this journey with him now and he is peeling away our infections and damage, one layer at a time. My son is healthy and improving in all areas. I am also improving and show few of the symptoms I used to have. The good news is that our doctor is now going to begin training other doctors on his methods. This way, more people across the country can benefit.

The LIA Foundation has flourished into an organization that is leading in information on the connection between Lyme disease, co-infections, and autism spectrum disorder. At just eight months old, we held our first conference in Southern California in which over 200 people came from all over the United States and Canada. In addition, a physicians' training course trained over forty physicians on different treatment options available to help our children. We plan to continue on this mission until we have made a difference and these children and parents are healed.

As for Michael, I can say with certainty now that my son is in recovery. He is not recovered. But we can touch it, and I can see in him the boy and man that he can and will be some day. He would make a great pastor, sales executive, scientist, dog trainer, or whatever he sets his mind to be. There is hope; my son is healing.

Research is finding that many tick and flea-borne infections infect untold thousands of children. These infections, such as Lyme, Bartonella, Babesia and Mycoplasma, are transmitted painlessly by invisible deer ticks, some vaccines, congenital transfer, or mere insect feces. Many cutting-edge scientists and physicians see this massive flood of emerging stealth infections and are publishing information about them. However, most physicians are obviously rushing through appointments, working merely to survive, and have little time for so much new information.

I tell you my story to give you a ray of hope. As parents, we need to look at every single possibility when it comes to our kids, even if our doctors are too busy to do so. Are you going to ignore the Lyme disease connection because it sounds off-the-wall? What if your child has it and you missed it? As you can see, children can heal even when they are a bit older. Our kids are worth it, and so are you.

BRYAN'S PREFACE: THE LYME-AUTISM CONNECTION CLOSE TO HOME

Some authors have a clinical, sterile, impersonal relationship with the content they write. My relationship with this book is quite the opposite. As an author, my personal experience with both Lyme disease and autism has been the driving force behind my desire to write this book. When I was about twenty-three years old, I had a friend who worked with autistic children at a middle school in the city where I grew up. I visited her during the workday, and I had a lot of contact with the autistic children.

Around the same time, I was diagnosed with Lyme disease. As time passed and I began to intensively study the disease, I became more and more intrigued by the autistic children at the middle school. Something told me—some underlying, gut instinct—that somehow, some way, these children had a disease similar to what I was suffering from. I had no way of proving this hunch. It just seemed that they were feeling what I was feeling.

Eventually, I lost contact with the autistic children of that local middle school. In the years that passed after my time with them, I would occasionally encounter a desperate mother of an autistic child, be her a family friend, distant relative, or just an acquaintance. The nagging instinct that I was somehow connected to these children would surface again for a few days, during which time I would ponder a possible Lyme-autism connection. This was back in approximately 2001, before I had heard about the connection. So, my initial thoughts on the topic were not sparked by a newspaper article or website, but were instead much more personal—a gut level, instinctual feeling.

In 2006, working as a professional healthcare journalist, I became acquainted with Tami Duncan, co-founder of the LIA Foundation. My forgotten experiences with autistic children and gut feeling about a possible connection between Lyme disease and autism dramatically resurfaced as I began to communicate with Tami. Sure enough, it appeared there actually was such a connection, even to the extent that annual conferences on the subject were taking place, bringing together some of the most credible and well-respected physicians in the Lyme and autism fields.

Although various articles and statements of hypotheses on the connection had been written, there was not a book on the topic. So, I undertook the project with Tami. As I embarked down the road of the hundreds of hours of research necessary for the book, I learned that the Lyme-autism connection was indeed much more than a hunch. It became obvious that this connection is supported by a great deal of science and the personal experiences of hundreds of mothers with autistic children. As I wrote the book and collaborated closely with Tami, I found that the central ideas and concepts were so fascinating and important that they practically leapt out of the research materials. This book needed to be written so badly that it practically wrote itself.

Looking back, I now realize that I have probably had Lyme disease since birth. I had experienced strange symptoms as a baby, and on into childhood (according to my parents). I spent the first three days of my life in intensive care, with a fever, apart from my mother and father. During my early teenage years, I always had aches, pains, migraine headaches, food intolerances, severe allergies, and mood swings. I just assumed that these symptoms were normal—"growing pains," my doctors said. When these same symptoms became debilitating in my early twenties, I knew they were not normal. They turned out to be a raging case of Lyme disease. They improved only after antibacterial treatment.

Perhaps, under slightly different circumstances, I myself may have ended up with autism. My symptoms began at birth. What really separated me from autistic children? Maybe a lot less than I would like to believe. After researching the Lyme-autism connection for months, I now believe that I was much closer to acquiring a severe developmental disorder than I had ever guessed or imagined.

As I write this, I am now a new father. I have a healthy, thriving nine-month old son. So far, he appears to be completely free of the health problems which changed the course of his father's life. However, I cannot count the number of nights I lost sleep during my wife's pregnancy, hoping and praying that my unborn child would be healthy. Although my wife is healthy and Lyme-free, recent research has shown that Lyme disease can be transmitted sexually, and also from mother to child during pregnancy. Did I give my wife a subclinical Lyme disease infection which might have been passed to my unborn child? So far, it appears we are in the clear. Yet, the potential guilt and dread of knowing I might have been responsible for adversely affecting both my wife and my child, has never escaped me.

Because of the current research being published, we have not vaccinated our son yet, and we are not sure whether or not we will vaccinate him in the future. I believe that some vaccines are dangerous enough *without* Lyme disease in the family history. When you add Lyme disease to the mix, the situation becomes even more precarious. It is now believed that Lyme disease and childhood vaccinations can act synergistically to create mayhem in the body. While one or the other may be merely dangerous, when combined, the two factors can become devastating.

Today, I am optimistic. Modern research and awareness is opening the doors to new treatments, effective prevention programs, and a deeper understanding of the complex web that is Lyme disease and autism. The dark ages are giving way to a new era which will bring health and hope to thousands of families.

Join me in the fight to discover and expose objective scientific truth, whatever that truth may be. Whether they be financial interests, political agendas, or simply the slow turning of the wheel of medical progress, together we can conquer all of the obstacles in the way of the health of our children. Human progress is dependent upon health, and health, I believe, is dependent upon honest, direct, and revealing journalism. The urgency of the situation, my passion for uncovering and exploring this connection, and the expertise brought to the table by those who contributed to this project, have culminated in a book which I hope you find as fascinating as I do.

Chapter 1
Introduction

The Twin Epidemics

A mother of three autistic children once made the following profound observation:

> *"Childhood autism has become so prevalent that there are very few who do not know of a family with an autistic child. Families with two autistic children are not uncommon, and I personally have seen a family in which all three of the family's children were autistic (very much like mine).*
>
> *The latest statistics estimate that over one half million American children are autistic, and with numbers steadily growing, there is no end in sight.*
>
> *It can be expected that treatments will improve the outlook of these children, but many or most of them will require custodial care for life, at an average cost to society of as much as three million dollars per child. Something must be stirring this explosive epidemic on, and one of the factors which has been greatly overlooked is the Lyme-autism connection."*
>
> —Kathy Blanco, mother of 3 autistic children and one of the original parents to discover the Lyme-autism connection

Over the last decade, two disease epidemics have gone from mild ripples in the water to roaring, ravenous, all-consuming tidal waves, destroying thousands of lives and tearing apart countless families.

These two diseases are Lyme disease and autism. Until recently, these afflictions were believed to be unrelated. Actually, that is an understatement. They were believed to have absolutely nothing in common, occupying distinct and opposite positions in the medical field. Whereas bronchitis and strep throat have some relationship in that they are both infections, Lyme disease and autism were thought to have nothing in common at all—one is a tick-borne infection which healthy people contract while camping, and the other is a prenatal brain development disorder. Recently, however, science has found similarities between Lyme disease and autism that cannot be ignored. When one looks beneath the surface of these seemingly diverse disorders, the underlying discoveries are shocking.

How did a possible connection between Lyme disease and autism become apparent? The connection hypothesis began, first and foremost, as a result of observant parents and physicians who noticed various undeniable, yet subtle, similarities between Lyme disease and autism.

For example, why have cases of autism skyrocketed over the past couple of decades? If autism is a genetic disorder, as it has been previously believed, how could such a rapid increase occur? Genetic disorders rarely involve such non-linear, exponential explosions in occurrence. Genes just don't change that fast. Infectious epidemics, on the other hand, such as Lyme disease, can and do cause exponential increases in disease cases. Also, why do the cases of autism continue to skyrocket even after mercury has been taken out of vaccines, and even in children who were never vaccinated?

Later in the book you'll read about statistics which show a strong correlation between the rising incidence of autism and the rising incidence of Lyme disease from 1992 to 2006. You will also read about a significant correlation between the geographic distribution of autism and Lyme disease cases. This data alone is enough to raise eyebrows.

Of course, mere statistical *correlation* between the incidence and distribution of Lyme disease and autism is not enough to use as a foundation for *causation*. If you recall your college statistics class, correlation does not necessarily imply causation. For example, morning traffic congestion is highly correlated with the time of day when the sun rises, because everyone drives to work early in the morning. There is a *correlation* between sunrise and rush hour traffic. Yet, rush hour traffic does not *cause* the sun to rise any more than sunrise itself causes people to get in their vehicles and go to work. Obviously, it is important to make the distinction between *correlation* and *causation*.

However, when the strong, but not necessarily conclusive, correlations between autism data and Lyme disease data are combined with other factors such as symptomology, epidemiology, family history, and the other factors that we will explore in this book, a very strong argument can be built for the case that similarities between Lyme disease and autism move beyond the realm of *correlation* into the territory of *causation*.

For these reasons, the Lyme-autism connection is rapidly gaining momentum and public awareness. Well-respected researchers, physicians, and organizations are beginning to take a second look at what might be the biggest infectious disease discovery of the century.

The Lyme-autism connection should not be surprising. For years, doctors and patients have noticed the similarities between Lyme disease and autism. Interestingly, Lyme disease often causes the most serious devastation in children. Consider this excerpt from a press release dated August 25, 2003, published by ILADS (International Lyme and Associated Diseases Society):

> *According to Robert Bransfield, MD, of New Jersey, "Lyme disease often strikes entire families and the result is a higher incidence of divorce, family dysfunction, and domestic violence. Patients are less able to think things through, and tend to act impulsively. A mother may suddenly lash out at her child and a husband may lose control and abuse his wife."*
>
> *Bransfield says young people are the most likely to act out. "I've seen so many straight-A kids whose grades suddenly start to slip. Then they rebel against the family and start fighting with their peers. However, these kids generally improve after treatment with antibiotics."*

Recognizing Lyme disease as a possible contributing factor in childhood developmental disorders is extremely important and urgent. Why? Since Lyme disease is currently an epidemic, with vastly increasing prevalence, if this causative factor in autism were missed, it could be expected that the number of cases of autism would continue to increase exponentially, in proportion to the number of cases of Lyme disease. Similarly, since autism is not the only disorder which Lyme disease can potentially induce, the incidence of other childhood disorders would also be expected to rise dramatically. On the other hand, if this causative factor is recognized, an incalculable amount of pain and suffering might be avoided by appropriately addressing Lyme disease in the prevention and treatment of autism and related childhood developmental disorders.

To date, we have observed a situation in which cases of autism and other childhood developmental disorders are, in fact, increasing roughly in proportion to cases of Lyme disease (see Chapter 6 for a complete statistical analysis). Hopefully, the information in this book will help curb this rise, as awareness increases and physicians and researchers begin to explore the Lyme-autism connection.

An Uphill Battle

Many people believe that objective scientific rules are used to classify diseases. You may be shocked to learn that the distinction between Lyme disease and autism (and numerous other "unrelated" diseases) as separate medical conditions is not a result of science alone, but also politics. Medical politics contributes to the unnatural and unscientific separation of many diseases into arbitrary categories, and hence, even if there actually were a Lyme-autism connection, it would be exceedingly difficult to identify due to the way modern medicine is organized. In other words, from the outset of our study into the Lyme-autism connection, we are facing an uphill battle, not only in discovering new scientific principles, but also in moving against the very fundamentals of modern medical practice.

Medical schools of thought in other countries, such as China, take a more holistic approach to classifying disease, viewing the body as an aggregate of interlinking systems. Western medicine, on the other hand, classifies and files away each cell, tissue, and organ in its own separate filing cabinet.

You have only to look in the phone book to see this separation. Flip open your local phone book to the "Physicians" section. If you have a problem with your teeth, you can find a dentist. If you have a problem with your heart, you can see a cardiologist. If you have a problem with your knee, you can make an appointment with an orthopedist. If you have a problem with your brain, you can dial up a neurologist, unless it is a psychological problem, in which case you can see a psychologist or psychiatrist.

The practice of separating health problems into "medical specialties" has advantages and disadvantages. Among the advantages is the fact that the specialist you pick out of the phone book will probably know more about your knee (or fill-in-the-blank body part) than any other doctor in your city. Among the disadvantages is the fact that if your knee problem is caused by arthritis, which is a problem of the immune system, you may end up undergoing unnecessary surgery as your orthopedic knee specialist does what he was trained to do: surgery on knees, completely ignoring the potential inter-connectedness of knees with other body systems, namely, the immune system.

Orthopedic knee specialists rarely communicate with immunologists, and in medical school, immunology classes rarely overlap with orthopedic classes, even though the health afflictions which both disciplines deal with can have a great deal of overlap (e.g., arthritis of the knee). Similarly, neurologists rarely communicate with psychologists, even though many neurological diseases, such as obsessive compulsive disorder, schizophrenia, and depression, can have root causes originating in both the biochemical realm as well as the behavioral-social realm.

The very act of discovering connections between supposedly unrelated conditions, given this paradigm of separation that governs modern medicine, is highly difficult, unlikely, and directly opposed by the modern organization and flow of medical information, funding, politics, and academics. Over the course of history, discoveries of connections between two supposedly unrelated illnesses have been vehemently opposed and denied before finally and reluctantly being accepted.

Take, for example, the connection between H. pylori bacteria and stomach ulcers. The scientists who discovered this connection were ridiculed and the association was not accepted until over a century had passed from the time the first discovery was made. In 1875, G. Bottcher and M. Letulle hypothesized that ulcers are caused by bacteria. In 1881, a scientist named Edwin Klebs noticed bacteria in the tissue of the human stomach. In 1939, A.

Stone Freedberg conducted a study and found H. pylori in the stomach lining, yet his colleagues denied the findings. It was not until 2005 that scientists named Warren and Marshall were given the Nobel Prize for their "discovery" of H. pylori as a cause of stomach ulcers. You can do the math: it took more than 100 years for the connection to be accepted.

And what about the connection between mercury poisoning and neurological disorders? Decades of scientific research supporting the connection was ignored and it took years until the majority of dentists stopped using amalgam in tooth repair products. And to this day, some dentists still use amalgam! Because of the compartmentalization that dictates disease classification and the resultant dogmatic specialization, connections between diseases are rarely unveiled, and when unveiled, they are slow to be accepted. The irrationality and blindness regarding these connections is captured eloquently in the first chapter of an excellent book by Andrew Hall Cutler, Ph.D., entitled *Amalgam Illness: Diagnosis and Treatment*. The following excerpt reveals how the "compartmentalization paradigm" can lead the government to take some very absurd actions:

> *"Vaccines and other injectables preserved with thimerosal, topical antiseptics and eye care products (recently taken off the market), and amalgam fillings expose people to mercury. There are an extremely large number of other sources of mercury exposure used in the medical industry. Sources of elemental mercury such as fluorescent lamps, thermometers, etc. are in theory recognized as hazards but in practice are treated very casually and do lead to poisoning when the mercury in them is not properly collected and disposed of.*

> *Now of course some government dweeb will try to tell you Andrew Cutler obviously doesn't know any chemistry—he must not have listened in those years and years of classes he took. Once the mercury is mixed up with silver in amalgam, it becomes perfectly safe! But in fact, it doesn't. Mercury has a certain vapor pressure. Mixing it up with another metal to make amalgam reduces the vapor pressure. Amalgam is comprised of half mercury, so the vapor pressure of mercury in the amalgam is about half that of regular*

mercury. Doesn't matter if it is solid or liquid. Solids evaporate just fine. How do you think the ice cubes in your freezer go away if you leave them for a long time, or all that fluffy white frost forms?

So here we have the government dweeb telling you out of one side of his mouth that you have to pay a zillion dollars to a hazardous waste disposal company to wear what amounts to spacesuits for the hour or two it takes them to clean up a mercury spill when they break a blood pressure meter in a doctor's office since it is SOOOOOOOO toxic and evaporates SOOOOOOO fast, and then telling you out of the other side of his mouth that it is perfectly fine to permanently install something half that toxic in your mouth without taking any precautions at all! Which side of his mouth do you believe?"

-From *Amalgam Illness: Diagnosis and Treatment*
Book available from www.lymebook.com/mercury

"So what?" you may be thinking. So American medicine is specialized and compartmentalized, even to an irrational extreme—why should you care? You should care because this specialization may be preventing your autistic child from receiving the best medical care. Autism is a multi-systemic, complicated disease. If there is a connection between Lyme disease and autism, your physicians will likely never discover it. The infectious disease doctor you are seeing was not trained to think about autism, and the autism specialist you are seeing was not trained to think about infectious diseases. These medical professionals specialize in the narrow cross-section of medicine in which they are board certified and practice, and they rarely venture into the fields of other physicians, let alone connect pathological disease processes to diagnoses which are outside of their training.

This "blind spot" for connections between seemingly unrelated diseases is not the fault of any specific physician or university. Instead, it is simply the result of years of momentum in the current medical paradigm. Nevertheless, before reading this book, you should know that your journey to discover the root cause of your child's autism will be an uphill battle as long as the medical system operates as it does. You will be the one—instead of your doctors—who needs to ask the hard questions and make the difficult connections, placing each puzzle piece on the table until you have the full puzzle.

If there is a connection between Lyme disease and autism, and if the science unquestionably supports such a connection, it will still likely be years, or maybe even decades, before mainstream medicine recognizes and accepts the connection. You will need to be your own advocate and demand the medical care that will take you down the road of healing. You don't have time to wait until the sluggish wheel of mainstream medicine turns over in the next 100 years. In the same way that you would demand your tab to be recalculated at a restaurant if a mistake were made, you must also demand that your inner circle of health care resources—e.g., your doctors, consultants, nurses, insurance companies, and support groups—face the facts and do their homework.

But even if a connection is uncovered and accepted, we face an even more challenging situation because numerous connections are involved in autism—hence, the "many faces" of autism...

The Many Faces of Autism

Western medicine, in its endless desire to methodically classify and distinguish modern health problems, has searched tirelessly for "the" cause of autism. The mainstream medical establishment is slow to recognize the multi-faceted nature of modern diseases, preferring instead the singular, tunnel-vision model of "only one cause per disease." Such tunnel vision is applied to the many common diseases of our time, including heart disease, high blood pressure, Alzheimer's, and multiple sclerosis.

With autism, the idea of a singular cause has contributed to much suffering, elusiveness in the study of autism, and difficulty in preventing and treating autism. The failure to recognize the multiplicity of causes that likely lead to autism results in missed research opportunities and a false understanding of the disease. One child may develop autism due to genetic factors, another may develop the disease as a result of vaccination, and yet a third may have been the victim of maternal substance abuse. Yet others may be the victims of infections such as Lyme disease. And any number of the above scenarios can also be mixed and matched under various circumstances.

Although painstakingly slow, mainstream medicine is showing hints that it is beginning to see the cracks in its classification system. Recently, in direct opposition to the predominant paradigm that separates health problems from each other and ignores the holistic picture, the National Institutes of Health (NIH), through which most government-funded medical research takes place, began painting autism in a new light. In September of 2006, *NIH News* published an article that admits the possibility that autism may have multiple causes. The article goes even further and states that "scientists are considering the likelihood of 'autisms,' that is, multiple disorders that comprise autism." According to the article, "Children with regressive autism appear to develop normal language and social skills but then lose these with the onset of autism before age 3. Non-regressive autism, the more common form of the disorder, begins early in life, possibly before birth, with evidence of subtle deficits throughout development." Although it will be years or decades before these views are integrated at the clinical level, we can be encouraged by the progress that is taking place.

Regardless of when the government (and hence, mainstream medicine) accepts the present realities, we can be sure of several facts. Since autism was first given its name by Hans Asperger in 1938, numerous causes have been studied and implicated in the development of the disorder. Although we still do not know with certainty what causes autism, we can be sure that it is more than one contributing factor, and we even know many of the culprits. Factors such as genetics, mercury from vaccinations, maternal health and substance abuse, environmental toxins, and infec-tions have been named over the years as possible—and some, already proven—contributors. It has been objectively proven that autistic children have been helped by treatments that are used to address a wide variety of health disorders. Yet, we ob-viously do not have the entire picture. If we did, we could cure autism.

Numerous researchers have described the multi-factorial nature of autism. Published in 1988, *Diagnosis and Assessment in Autism,* edited by Eric Schopler and Gary B. Mesibov, offers the following observation: "It is clear that the preponderance of available evidence suggests the importance of multiple biologic factors acting through one or more mechanisms to produce the autistic syndrome." This is only one example of dozens of books, articles, studies and publications that describe the broad range of potential causative factors in autism.

So where does Lyme disease fit in? This book does not claim that Lyme disease is "the" cause of autism. Such a claim would be scientifically unfounded. However, what this book does do is present a scientifically backed argument that Lyme disease may be one of the contributing factors involved in the development of the disease. Intentionally avoiding the tunnel vision mentality, this book presents the Lyme-autism connection as one piece of the puzzle, not the whole puzzle.

While it is clear that Lyme disease is not *the* cause of autism, the Lyme disease puzzle piece may in fact help explain why the other factors fit into the puzzle where they do. Take vaccines, for ex-ample. The correlation between autism and vaccine-induced damage is well established, albeit not completely understood. The presence of the Lyme disease infection in an autistic child may help to explain why vaccinations have the effect that they do. An article by Tony Edwards, published in a publication called

What Doctors Don't Tell You, sheds further light on the puzzle—
here is an excerpt:

> *Of course, scores of theories have been proposed for the cause of*
> *autism, among which vaccine damage is perhaps the best known.*
> *But Lyme disease may be involved there, too. "It is possible that the*
> *two [Lyme disease and autism] are conjoined in damage, and the*
> *long-term effects of Borrelia could hamper the body's ability to*
> *mount a significant, timely response to vaccines," says Dr Geoffrey*
> *Radoff, of the Alternative Medical Care Center of Arizona. "This*
> *could explain the higher incidences of adverse reactions to*
> *vaccinations in children with autism (Townsend Letter for Doctors*
> *and Patients, April, 2007).*

In addition, the opposite scenario may occur: Instead of Lyme
disease preventing an adequate response to vaccinations, the
vaccines themselves may hinder the body's ability to ward off a
Lyme infection. Although most vaccinations are now mercury-
free, this has not always been the case. Thimerosal (mercury)
was once widely used as a preservative in vaccines. It is well
established that mercury is immuno-suppressive and greatly
hinders the body's ability to fight Lyme disease and other infections. In fact, as I (Bryan) explain in my recently published book,
The Top 10 Lyme Disease Treatments, Lyme bacteria may actually sequester mercury and use it in an effort to weaken the
host immune response and create a toxic, protective niche in the
body. Furthermore, many of the other ingredients in vaccines are
also immunosuppressive, leading to a possible weakening of the
body's ability to fight infections such as Lyme. So, as you can see,
many of the pieces of the puzzle are interrelated. Vaccinations
and Lyme disease, while separate pieces, may, in fact, be synergistic factors in the development of autism.

As the inevitable truth of autism as a multi-factorial disease
permeates modern science, the mainstream media is beginning
to pick up the story (even before the government and large university medical schools do). In an article released on April 1,
2008, entitled, *Tracing Autism's Roots*, CNN.com reported that

"environmental factors may conspire with predisposing genes to bring on autism." This article, which cited genetics as the primary culprit in autism, also made some other interesting state-statements. If indeed autism is passed on genetically, then an infectious root cause such as Lyme disease would be less likely (Lyme disease, while possibly passed from mother to child during pregnancy, is not passed down through multiple generations in the same way that genes are). The article notes, however, the following new finding with regard to the genetic predisposition:

"There is a new wrinkle to the genetic research however. Based on family studies, scientists have long characterized autism-linked genes as "heritable." But recent research shows a surprisingly large number of mutations tied to autism are "de novo" glitches that arise spontaneously in children whose parents don't carry them."

What? Stop for a second. This is a powerful statement. The gene chain believed to confer autism is, for some reason, broken in some cases. This sets the stage for some type of extraneous, spontaneous, one-time insult to the developing child—such as an infection. In fact, this CNN.com article, which received widespread distribution and viewership, even went as far as to implicate potential infectious causes:

"For all geneticists' excitement...few if any of them rule out environmental contributors to autism, such as exposure to certain drugs, chemicals or infections during pregnancy...environmental factors may conspire with predisposing genes to bring on autism."

Figure 1 (next page), which was created by Jeffrey Wulfman, MD, offers a graphical depiction of the many factors which can lead to autism.

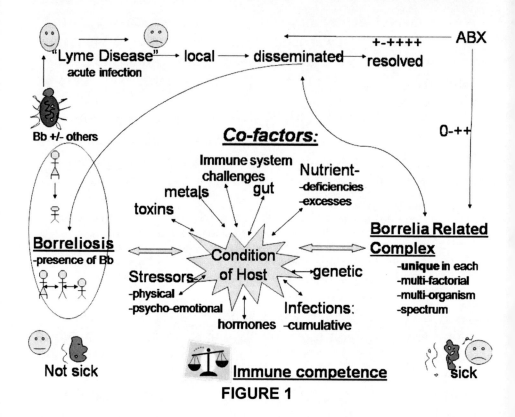

FIGURE 1

CNN.com (and also this book) makes it known that autism is multi-factorial, and likely has more than one cause. Nevertheless, as the CNN.com article points out, there are some strange and unexpected twists in the plot—namely, a break in the gene pattern and the possibility of infectious origin—which leave room for the Lyme-autism hypothesis.

In addressing the multi-faceted nature of autism, Garth Nicolson, Ph.D., of the Institute for Molecular Medicine, presented the following at the 2007 LIA Foundation conference:

Possible roles of chronic infections in autism:

1. Chronic infections (bacterial, viral, fungal) could be the cause of the illness.

2. Chronic infections could be a co-factor with other factors (chemical, heavy metals, etc.) as the cause of illness.

3. Chronic infections could be opportunistic and occur after immune suppression.

4. Chronic infections could cause co-morbid states in chronic illness.

In addition to autism, many other childhood developmental disorders, including Attention Deficit Disorder, Asperger's syndrome, PDD-NOS (Pervasive Developmental Disorder - Not Otherwise Specified), also appear to involve infectious etiology. While this book focuses specifically on autism, it should be understood that just as Lyme disease can manifest in so many seemingly unrelated symptom complexes in adults (such as chronic fatigue syndrome, fibromyalgia, arthritis, schizophrenia, obsessive compulsive disorder, multiple sclerosis, Alzheimer's disease, Parkinson's, etc—see Appendix B for more), it can do the same in children.

The Lyme-autism connection extends far beyond just autism to encompass many (maybe even dozens) of other childhood and adult diseases. The ramifications of this wide-reaching fact are numerous. If we can figure out how to deal with Lyme disease in autism, maybe we can also figure out how to deal with it in dozens of other illnesses and potentially hundreds of thousands of chronically sick people.

But Isn't Lyme disease Just a Simple Bacteria?

Maybe you are wondering how Lyme disease could possibly be one of the root causes of autism. Isn't Lyme disease just a simple bacterial infection acquired from a tick bite? Can't it be cured with 10 days of antibiotics? Aren't the symptoms fairly simple, such as inflamed joints, fever, and headache? How can such a simple disease be involved in autism, which is a complex, chronic, multi-systemic, neurological disease?

The answers to these questions may shock you and may be the opposite of what you had guessed. The truth about the complexity and severity of Lyme disease is unbeknownst to most people. This topic will be addressed in detail in the chapters of this book. In this section, however, for the purpose of introducing you to the intricacies of chronic Lyme disease, we will present a list of facts about Lyme disease produced by ILADS (International Lyme and Associated Diseases Society, www.ILADS.org). This list is eye-opening and will help you begin to understand the reality of the threat that Lyme disease poses. Although the list does not encompass all of the relevant complexities—additional complexities appear in context throughout this book—it will give you a framework upon which to base your understanding of and appreciation for the seriousness of Lyme disease.

ILADS List: Basic Information about Lyme Disease

1. Lyme disease is transmitted by the bite of a tick, and the disease is **prevalent across the United States and throughout the world**. Ticks know no borders and respect no boundaries. A patient's county of residence does not accurately reflect his or her Lyme disease risk because people travel, pets travel, and ticks travel.

This creates a dynamic situation with many opportunities for exposure to Lyme disease for each individual.

2. Lyme disease is a **clinical diagnosis**. The disease is caused by a spiral-shaped bacteria (spirochete) called *Borrelia burgdorferi*. The Lyme spirochete can cause infection of multiple organs and produce a wide range of symptoms. Case reports in the medical literature document the protean manifestations of Lyme disease, and familiarity with its varied presentations is key to recognizing disseminated disease.

3. **Fewer than 50%** of patients with Lyme disease recall a **tick bite**. In some studies this number is as low as 15% in culture-proven infection with the Lyme spirochete.

4. **Fewer than 50%** of patients with Lyme disease recall any rash. Although the erythema migrans (EM) or "bull's-eye" rash is considered classic, it is not the most common dermatologic manifestation of early-localized Lyme infection. Atypical forms of this rash are seen far more commonly. It is important to know that the EM rash is pathognomonic of Lyme disease and requires no further verification prior to starting an appropriate course of antibiotic therapy.

5. The Centers for Disease Control and Prevention (CDC) **surveillance** criteria for Lyme disease were devised to track a narrow band of cases for epidemiologic purposes. As stated on the CDC website, the surveillance criteria were **never** intended to be used as diagnostic criteria, nor were they meant to define the entire scope of Lyme disease.

6. The **ELISA** screening test is unreliable. The test **misses 35%** of culture proven Lyme disease (only 65% sensitivity) and is unacceptable as the first step of a two-step screening protocol. By definition, a screening test should have at least 95% sensitivity.

7. Of patients with acute culture-proven Lyme disease, **20–30% remain seronegative** on serial **Western Blot** sampling. Antibody titers also appear to decline over time; thus while the Western Blot may remain positive for months, it may not always be sensitive enough to detect chronic infection with the Lyme spirochete. For "epidemiological purposes" the CDC eliminated from the Western Blot analysis the reading of **bands 31 and 34**. These bands are so specific to *Borrelia burgdorferi* that they were chosen for vaccine development. Since a vaccine for Lyme disease is currently unavailable, however, a positive 31 or 34 band is highly indicative of *Borrelia burgdorferi* exposure. Yet these bands are not reported in commercial Lyme tests.

8. When used as part of a diagnostic evaluation for Lyme disease, the Western Blot should be performed by a **laboratory that reads and reports all of the bands** related to *Borrelia burgdorferi*. Laboratories that use FDA approved kits (for instance, the Mardx Marblot®) are restricted from reporting all of the bands, as they must abide by the rules of the manufacturer. These rules are set up in accordance with the CDCs surveillance criteria and increase the risk of false-negative results. The commercial kits may be useful for surveillance purposes, but they offer too little information to be useful in patient management.

9. There are 5 subspecies of *Borrelia burgdorferi*, **over 100 strains in the US**, and 300 strains worldwide. This diversity is thought to contribute to the antigenic variability of the spirochete and its ability to evade the immune system and antibiotic therapy, leading to chronic infection.

10. Testing for *Babesia, Anaplasma, Ehrlichia* and *Bartonella* (other tick-transmitted organisms) should be performed. The presence of **co-infection** with these organisms points to probable infection with the Lyme spirochete as well. If these coinfections are left

untreated, their continued presence **increases morbidity** and prevents successful treatment of Lyme disease.[1]

11. A preponderance of evidence indicates that **active ongoing spirochetal infection** with or without other tick-borne coinfections is the **cause of the persistent symptoms in chronic Lyme disease.**

12. **There has never been a study demonstrating that 30 days of antibiotic treatment cures chronic Lyme disease.** However there is a plethora of documentation in the US and European medical literature demonstrating by histology and culture techniques that short courses of antibiotic treatment fail to eradicate the Lyme spirochete. Short treatment courses have resulted in upwards of a 40% relapse rate, especially if treatment is delayed.

13. Most cases of chronic Lyme disease require an extended course of antibiotic therapy to achieve symptomatic relief. The return of symptoms and evidence of the continued presence of *Borrelia burgdorferi* indicates the need for further treatment. The very **real consequences of untreated chronic persistent Lyme infection** far outweigh the potential consequences of long-term antibiotic therapy.

14. Many patients with chronic Lyme disease require treatment for 1–4 years, or until the patient is symptom-free. Relapses occur and maintenance antibiotics may be required. There are no tests currently available to prove that the organism is eradicated or that the patient with chronic Lyme disease is cured.

---

[1] Current testing for these organisms is vastly inadequate. In Dr. James Schaller's two extensive textbooks, *The Diagnosis and Treatment of Babesia* and *The Diagnosis and Treatment of Bartonella*, he reports that routine testing at the larger national labs for both infections is grossly flawed. For example, after sending many samples of malaria-like Babesia to be examined closely and specifically for "malaria or Babesia," these large labs have yet to report obvious Babesia clearly present inside red blood cells in large numbers.

15. Like Syphilis in the 19th century, Lyme disease has been called the **great imitator** and should be considered in the differential diagnosis of rheumatologic and neurologic conditions, as well as chronic fatigue syndrome, fibromyalgia, somatization disorder and any difficult-to-diagnose multi-system illness.

16. **ILADS Disclaimer:** The foregoing information is **for educational purposes only**. It is not intended to replace or supersede patient care by a healthcare provider. If an individual suspects the presence of a tick-borne illness, that individual should consult a healthcare provider who is familiar with the diagnosis and treatment of tick-borne diseases.

See Appendix B for more introductory information on Lyme disease. It is absolutely critical that you understand that Lyme disease is anything but a simple bacterial infection. It is highly complex and mimics dozens of seemingly unrelated mental illnesses.

Infection Stew

We have seen that there are many potential causes, or many faces, of autism, one of which is infections. To make the situation even more complicated, the category of infections must itself be broken down into sub-categories. When this book describes a possible connection between autism and Lyme disease, what we are really referring to is a connection between autism and the dozens of infections, including fungi, bacteria, and viruses, that comprise the Lyme disease "infectious stew."

You may be surprised to learn that, in most cases, the Lyme disease infection (caused by bacteria called Borrelia burgdorferi) is accompanied by other, partner infections. In the world of Lyme disease, LLMDs (Lyme Literate Medical Doctors) refer to the companion infections found with Lyme disease as "co-infections." These infections can include Babesia, Ehrlichia,

Bartonella, Mycoplasma, Anaplasma, and Candida, among dozens of others. If you are not already educated about Lyme disease, you may be surprised to learn that Lyme disease is not merely one bacterial infection, but a conglomeration of infections, all of which have devastating and synergistic effects.

There are a number of reasons why coinfections occur in conjunction with Lyme disease. The ticks which host Lyme disease bacteria are often hosts to dozens of other microorganisms. Hence, when a person is bitten by a tick, these other infections are typically passed along with it. However, even if a person becomes infected with only Borrelia burgdorferi, it is still probable that coinfections will enter the scene. Borrelia burgdorferi itself weakens the immune system and creates unhealthy bioterrain in which opportunistic, infectious microorganisms can thrive. So, once Borrelia burgdorferi is present, the door is opened for a plethora of other bacteria, fungi, parasites and viruses to enter.

The importance of recognizing this "infection stew" cannot be overstated. Suspecting, testing for, and treating coinfections is critical to successful healing. With regard to the Lyme-autism connection, the co-infection factor provides additional support for the connection hypothesis. Typically, when autistic children test positive for infections, they test positive for numerous infections, not merely a single infection. The same is true of Lyme disease patients.

In addition to the fact that multiple infections may contribute to autism, it is important to recognize that multiple infections may also be contributing to other childhood developmental disorders as well. Autism is not the only disease whose numbers are exploding across the United States. Numerous other childhood developmental disorders are skyrocketing as well, including, of particular note, Attention Deficit and Hyperactivity Disorder (ADHD).

The skyrocketing number of cases of ADHD is very telling for a number of reasons. First, if indeed autism can be caused by infections such as Lyme disease, it would follow that children of all ages, not just children younger than 36 months old (this is the average age for a diagnosis of autism) should be coming down with autism-like syndromes. Furthermore, adults should also be contracting similar syndromes. Why? Because Lyme disease bacteria, whether transmitted by an insect bite or another route of transmission, does not prefer any particular age, gender, race, or geography; the disease can strike anywhere, anytime. So, just as cases of autism are skyrocketing, we would also expect to see a rise in cases of similar diseases contracted later in life.

And indeed, this is happening. Although the symptoms and syndromes vary, diseases very similar to autism have been increasing in prevalence. Cases of child- and adult-onset ADHD are on the rise, in a similar fashion to the skyrocketing cases of Lyme disease itself as reported by the Centers for Disease Control and other regulatory agencies.

The NIDS (Neuro-Immune Dysfunction Syndromes) Medical Research Board, a coalition of parents and scientists who study the relationship between infections and behavioral disorders, sheds further light on this topic. The NIDS Board is comprised of the following physicians: Jeffrey Galpin, MD, Michael Goldberg, MD, Julie Griffith, MD, Nancy Klimas, MD, Ismael Mena, MD, Byron Hyde, MD, James Oleske, MD, and Vijendra Singh, PhD. According to their website, *"The NIDS Research Institute, which consists of the NIDS Parents Coalition and the NIDS Scientific Board, is dedicated to increasing the public's awareness of the likely connection between neuro-immune and/or auto-immune dysfunction and conditions such as Autism, ADD, Alzheimer's, ALS, CFS/CFIDS, MS, PDD and other immune-mediated diseas-*

es. *The Institute is also committed to facilitating access to treatment options and research studies for families suffering from these disease processes."*

A recent article by the NIDS Board, entitled *Clinical Hypothesis - Immune "Dysfunction / Dysregulation" - A Reason for Childhood Neuro-Cognitive Dysfunction,* began with the following statement:

> *"From an epidemiological standpoint, autism has migrated from a rare disorder to one that is now ten (10) to twenty (20) times more likely to be diagnosed. Ten years ago, "autism" occurred in 1-3 per 10,000 births. Now, current estimates suggest an incidence rate of 20-40 per 10,000 births. In fact, "cluster groups" throughout the world are currently being analyzed due to even higher incidence rates. It is also worth noting that other neuro-cognitive conditions such as "quiet" ADHD and "mixed" ADHD have received a renewed focus and attention among children and adolescents due to their perceived increase in incidence rates. Although a portion of these increases can likely be attributed to better and earlier recognition by the medical community and parents, the NIDS Board believes that this increase must prompt a change in how we approach these children. Specifically, we must begin to consider that these are not congenital, brain-damaged conditions but instead are medical disease processes acquired early in life."*

The NIDS medical hypothesis statement goes on to discuss forms of autism and ADHD which have a late onset, meaning that, before the disease struck, affected children were healthy and normal. This observation is important because it means that autism and ADHD, in many cases, are not entirely genetically-based, but instead, are triggered by an event in early life—a tick bite, possibly.

An obvious question arises at this point. Why would Lyme disease and associated infections affect babies differently than older children and adults, resulting in autism in the very young and ADHD in older people? There are numerous potential explanations for this, however, the primary explanation is simply that younger brains are more vulnerable to trauma and hence the syndrome that occurs when Lyme disease infects a young brain is more severe. ADHD may be a milder form of Lyme infection that takes hold of more mature brains, whereas autism may be a more severe form of Lyme infection that grips the newly developed, or developing, brains of infants and babies.

Still another question looms, and begs to be answered. If Lyme disease is passed to humans by the bite of an infected tick, how on earth can the infection possibly get inside a baby developing inside the womb? ADHD occurring in older children makes sense because older children can be exposed to ticks. But what about the unborn? We know that some cases of autism begin in the womb. How could Lyme disease possibly be involved?

This is the central question of the book you now hold in your hands. It is now believed that, in addition to tick bites, Lyme disease may also be transmitted in a number of other ways, including bites from other types of insects (such as flies, mosquitoes, and fleas), sexual contact, and transmission from mother to child during pregnancy. The latter will be the focus of Chapter 2, in which we will examine possible trans-placental transfer of the Lyme disease infection from mother to child during gestation.

On the Front Lines

Before heading into Chapter 2 and exploring the possibility that Lyme disease can be congenitally transferred, we would first like to share with you a brief, yet profound note from the founder of a cutting-edge integrative medicine clinic on the front lines of research and discovery in modern medicine.

In Austin, Texas, CARE Clinics (www.mycareclinics.com) was founded by Kazuko Curtin. Kazuko is the mother of a 13 year-old autistic boy—her firstborn.

Kazuko learned from an esteemed expert at The University of California, San Francisco (UCSF) that her son was a very low-functioning autistic child with no hope of recovery. After the diagnosis, Kazuko began the journey which eventually culminated in the founding of CARE Clinics. Kazuko believes the UCSF autism expert was wrong—she believes there is always hope.

According to the CARE Clinics website,

> *Autism, like many childhood afflictions whose incidences are rising, is a condition with biomedical underpinnings. It is not a behavioral disorder, although it has many behavioral disorder symptoms. It is a biomedical disorder. The problem to date has been that the biomedical aspects manifest themselves in as many ways as there are degrees "on the spectrum." People are looking for one answer, where instead autism has many—each child has their own answers. The key is to break the disease down, on an individual basis, into the specific parts for the particular child.*

> *The mainstream medical community, the AMA, the pediatricians and the medical researchers are all withholding opinion. It is the nature of our cautious system to perform endless clinical trials and double-blind studies. The legal system and the insurance systems are built this way to protect the public. This is great for children yet to be born, those that are two generations out. It does nothing however for my son, for the current generation of innocent children and families suffering under the tremendous physical, emotional and financial burdens of autism.*

> *At CARE Clinics we have studied the latest and greatest treatments for autism for the past eight years. As with all industries, politics and vested interests sometimes stifle progress. We believe the answer is in front of us and we are working with families who are interested in taking advantage of the latest advances in the treatment of autism as a disease with biomedical underpinnings. We are seeing great results by breaking the disease down into its modular parts, and then treating those parts.*

> *There is hope for our children and it gets brighter every day.*

In a recent conversation I (Bryan) had with Kazuko, I asked her about the Lyme disease test results of the children being cared for at CARE Clinics. Here is her response:

Lyme Induced Autism (LIA) Foundation: www.liafoundation.org

Dear Bryan,

Our children need so much help. Most health care professionals do not understand so many things. Sometimes, common sense should come before traditional, dogmatic approaches to medicine.

In the beginning, I believed that Lyme disease was not a big problem among the children at our clinic—I believed this because test markers (PCR and IgG) were negative. However, as the children get stronger and their immune systems begin to recover, and months pass, IgG markers begin getting higher and higher. Eventually, the Lyme infection is even detected by PCR. We have more than few cases like this to report.

We are currently working on formalizing our data. Hopefully we can report something significant in the near future. More research is needed.

Sincerely yours,

Kazuko
Founder
CARE Clinics
www.mycareclinics.com

What is so interesting about this note? Well, Kazuko's clinic is reporting a very fascinating finding. Since many types of Lyme disease tests detect the infection based on the body's own immune response to the infection, suppressed immunity in the patient can cause false-negative test results. What Kazuko is reporting here is that as the children at her clinic get stronger, and their immune systems recover, they are beginning to get positive test results for Lyme disease.

The fact that Lyme tests rely on a patient's immunity leads to a high number of false-negative tests in both adults and children, but especially in people with compromised immunity, such as those suffering from autism. "Negative test result," says the average physician, "means no Lyme disease." This might be one reason why certain autistic children test negative for Lyme.

Given what we know about the lack of reliability of Lyme disease tests, maybe some of these children actually do have Lyme disease. In fact, Kazuko's son was just diagnosed with CDC-positive Lyme disease one month before this book was published.

Maybe it is time to take a closer look at the Lyme-autism connection.

Chapter 2
Building the Foundation

Congenital Transfer

The first step in setting the stage for the Lyme-autism connection hypothesis is to ask whether or not Lyme disease can be passed from mother to child during pregnancy. This is the most important initial question because many cases of autism are thought to begin in the prenatal (inside the womb) phase of a child's life. If Lyme disease cannot be transferred inside the womb, then the Lyme-autism connection is, by definition, ruled out in many—if not most—cases of autism. In other words, the question of congenital transfer is the cornerstone of the foundation for the Lyme-autism connection.

In the words of Tami Duncan, printed in the June, 2008 issue of *Townsend Letter for Doctors and Patients,*

> *"Injecting babies with obscene amounts of thimerosal [mercury] can be blamed for triggering autistic symptoms in many children, but what can explain the susceptibility factor? Why did my child get autism, while your child didn't? Furthermore, why does autism occur in both vaccinated and non-vaccinated children of the same*

family? The answer could lie with the mothers...and infections may be the answer we need to solve this puzzle."

In the above-quoted article, Tami goes on to explain that many mothers of autistic children are themselves actually experiencing symptoms of chronic disease which might indicate an as-yet undetected Lyme infection. Could sick mothers be passing the Lyme infection on to their children? Or, because Lyme disease does not always cause active symptoms and may exist only at a subclinical level, perhaps asymptomatic, yet infected mothers may have Lyme disease and not even know it. Can a subclinical infection be passed on during pregnancy? These are the questions we will look at in this chapter.

You may be thinking, at this point, "Hold on a minute—you are telling me that as a mother, it may be my fault that my child has autism?" Well, that is sort of what we are telling you, although "fault" is not an accurate word to use. Of course you never *intended* to pass on any unwanted health problems to your child. However, it is no secret that parental health plays an important role in the health of our offspring. The most common example of this can be found in the genetics you pass on. Is your child a natural athlete? It may be a result of genetics. Numerous genetic diseases are well accepted by science. And, now, you might be able to add infections to the list of health conditions that may be conferred by innocent and loving parents. It is not your *fault*, but as a potential causative factor, it must be considered. Unraveling your own health problems may help you to isolate, analyze, and eventually heal *your child's* health problems.

This requires the introduction of a new paradigm—a new way of thinking about childhood disease—taking into consideration not just what happens to the baby, but also the mother. And in many ways this paradigm is not new at all, as it has long been known that a mother's actions while pregnant (whether intentional or accidental) can have consequences for the baby.

We are not yet asking the question of whether childhood onset Borreliosis (Lyme disease) leads to autism. We will save that question for later. Right now we are simply asking the foundational question of whether or not Lyme disease can be passed from mother to child during pregnancy. We will use the answer to this question as a premise for the Lyme-autism connection.

Throughout this chapter we will be looking at scientific research published recently as well as that which was published over the past several decades. Let's begin with a recent study, published in *The Journal of Neurotoxicology* in October of 2007. This study, conducted by UC Davis, was entitled "Autism: Maternally derived antibodies specific for fetal brain proteins" and found that,

> *"The presence of maternal autoantibodies to fetal brain proteins of approximately 37kDa and 73kDa molecular weight confers an elevated risk for autism...these data provide evidence for an association between the presence of maternal immune system biomarkers and a diagnosis of autism in a subset of children. The presence of specific anti-fetal antibodies in the circulation of mothers during pregnancy may be a potential trigger that, when paired with genetic susceptibility, is sufficient to induce a downstream effect on neurodevelopment leading to autism."*

In other words, your health as a mother can have an impact on your child. More specifically, the health of your immune system can have an impact on your child. In reference to the above, Robert Bransfield, MD, of Red Bank, New Jersey, provided information during his presentation at the April, 2007 LIA Foundation conference indicating that the above-mentioned 37kDa protein is associated with Borrelia burgdorferi, E.Coli, Bartonella, and Mycoplasma. The protein with a weight of 73kDa, according to Dr. Bransfield, is linked to Chlamydia, Strep, Mycoplasma, Bartonella, and also Borrelia burgdorferi.

Can a mother's health affect her children? The answer is unequivocally "yes." Let's now get more specific and ask, Can a mother's health affect her children if the mother is infected with Lyme disease bacteria—even if the mother is unaware of the infection?

We will now turn our attention to the life work and research of John Drulle, MD, who lived from 1944 to 2003. Dr. Drulle's work on Lyme disease was far before his time; this doctor made discoveries and announced findings about Lyme disease which were not recognized and adopted by the Lyme disease community until decades later, if at all. A mechanical engineer turned physician, Dr. Drulle had a creative and piercing ability to get to the bottom of difficult health challenges. To learn more about his work, visit the John Drulle Memorial Lyme Fund website at www.johndrullelymefund.org.

The foundation that bears Dr. Drulle's name granted us permission in the writing of this book to reproduce one of his most influential articles, entitled, *Pregnancy and Lyme Disease*, written in 1990 (notice that nearly two decades have passed since this information became available). In this article you will be escorted through numerous scientific studies—along with thoughtful analysis of those studies—relating to the congenital transfer of Lyme disease. Read what Dr. Drulle has written, and see for yourself what the scientific literature says.

PREGNANCY AND LYME DISEASE, BY JOHN DRULLE, MD

[Article written in 1990] When a pregnant woman is infected with Lyme disease, not only is she subject to its devastation, but her baby is too. At this time there is only a small amount of information available in the medical literature. I will review the major articles, and after describing our own experiences with

Lyme and pregnancy, present what I feel is a rational approach to this issue.

The first case of transplacental passage of Borrelia burgdorferi was reported in 1985 in Wisconsin by Schlesinger. The woman was bitten during her first trimester and developed an EM rash with two satellite lesions. This was followed by typical Lyme symptoms. She did not receive medical treatment as Lyme was not diagnosed at the time. She delivered a male baby at 35 weeks. The baby died 39 hours later from congestive heart failure, and at autopsy there were several major defects of the heart. Spirochetes were found in the spleen, kidneys, bone marrow and the heart. The mother tested positive for Lyme. Here we can only speculate that the Lyme might have been responsible for the birth defects, as these same types of problems can occur in non-Lyme situations.

In 1987, Dr. Alan MacDonald reported a case of a woman infected with Lyme in her first trimester of pregnancy, which unfortunately was not diagnosed or treated. She had developed a circular red rash which was followed by painful swelling of her knee. These resolved spontaneously. The woman went into labor at term, and delivered a 2,500 gram stillborn baby. Autopsy revealed a ventricular septal defect, i.e. a hole in the wall of the heart which separates the two main pumping chambers. The Lyme bacterium was cultured from the baby's liver, and it was demonstrated in the brain, heart, adrenal gland and the placenta. The mother's blood tested positive for antibodies to the Lyme spirochete and negative for Syphilis. Dr. MacDonald reported three other cases of fetal death in the second trimester, in which the Lyme spirochete was cultured from the livers. None of the mothers gave any history suggesting Lyme infection.

In 1986, Weber reported a case of Lyme infection in a newborn baby. The mother had been bitten by multiple ticks during her first trimester. She developed an EM rash several weeks later. She was treated with a "standard" course of oral penicillin for seven days, three times a day. The baby was delivered at term and appeared normal. During the next 23 hours the baby developed breathing problems and died. Autopsy showed brain hemorrhages. Spirochetes compatible with Borrelia burgdorferi, the Lyme spirochete, were demonstrated in the brain and the liver. Initial testing of the mother's blood was negative for antibodies to the Lyme spirochete; however, at a later date her frozen blood tested positive for IgM antibodies by the ELISA test.

Markowitz published a study of Lyme and pregnancy in 1986. He described nineteen patients who were infected during pregnancy. Five of these had adverse outcomes (one fetal death at 20 weeks, high bilirubin level in a four-week premature baby, webbed toes, blindness and developmental delay, and a newborn rash). Thirteen of the nineteen had received antibiotics. The authors concluded that there was no proof that Lyme was responsible for the adverse outcomes since all of them were dissimilar. However, there was a consensus that this was an abnormally high frequency of adverse outcomes, and that pregnant women with diagnosed Lyme should be treated immediately with penicillin.

Williams and colleagues conducted a study of umbilical cord blood in a Lyme-endemic area in New York. Of 255 infants tested, 10.2% had detectable antibody to the Lyme spirochete. Of 166 infants born in a non-endemic area, 2.4% had detectable antibodies. The rate of birth defects did not differ significantly between the two groups; however, the first group tended to be of lower birth weight and smaller for their gestational age, and tended to have more jaundice. The authors concluded that these differences were not significantly different. A glaring flaw in this study is that it only included live births. Since miscarriages, stillbirth and perinatal infant deaths were not included, the possibility of congenital defects possibly associated with Lyme and incompatible with life are not included. Therefore, the authors' contention that no association exists between gestational Lyme and congenital defects should be viewed with a degree of skepticism.

Dr. Andrea Dlesk, of the Marshfield clinic in Wisconsin, studied 143 healthy pregnant women. Lyme serologic tests were obtained on the initial and postpartum visits. At the time the data were reported, 116 women had completed their pregnancies and 12 had miscarried, one of whom tested positive. Of the 104 women who did not miscarry, 13 women tested positive for Lyme. The conclusion was that healthy women who test positive for Lyme are at no increased risk for miscarriage. Again this study is flawed in that there are no autopsy data on the 12 miscarriages. It is quite possible that, in the 11 seronegative mothers who miscarried, seronegative Lyme was present and may have caused defective fetuses. Seronegative Lyme is a real entity and may account for 25% of all cases of Lyme.

In 1988, Carlomango studied 49 women who had either a 1st or 2nd trimester spontaneous abortion. Six (6) of them (12.2%) tested positive, compared to 3 of 49 women who delivered at term. The authors concluded that there was no statistical significance between the two groups.

In 1988, Nadal surveyed 1,416 women and their 1,434 infants at delivery for presence of antibodies to the Lyme spirochete. Twelve women tested positive (only one had a history compatible with EM during pregnancy), six had a history of pre-existing Lyme and five had unremarkable histories. Of these twelve women, seven had remarkable outcomes:

1. Two had elevated bilirubinemia

2. One had muscle hypotonia (laxness)

3. One was post-term, small for age, and evidenced chronic placental insufficiency

4. One had transient macrocephaly (large head)

5. One had transient supraventricular extrasystoles ("skipped heart beats")

6. The infant born of the mother with EM had a VSD-hole in the heart connecting the two main pumping chambers.

Since none of these babies had positive blood tests for antibodies to Lyme, the conclusion was that the adverse outcomes were not due to Lyme. The major flaw in this conclusion is the assumption that congenital Lyme babies are seropositive. This has been refuted by the work of Dr. Alan MacDonald, and is analogous to the findings of seronegativity in congenital Syphilis. [Note from Bryan Rosner: Recall from Chapter 1 Kazuko Curtin's experience at CARE Clinics with seronegative Lyme disease].

In 1989, Dr. Alan MacDonald reported his findings in autopsies performed following perinatal deaths at Southhampton Hospital between 1978 and 1988. It must be noted that routine pathology studies on tissues will not demonstrate the Lyme spirochete. Unless there is a high index of suspicion for Lyme disease, the special silver or immunologic stains which can identify the spirochete are not used. He also reports four cases where there was live birth and spirochetes were demonstrated in the placentas. In the group of perinatal deaths there was no history or evidence of Lyme disease in the mothers. Their blood tests were negative in all but one case. Spirochetes compatible with Borrelia burgdorferi were identified in the vital organs and numerous developmental defects were observed. Dr. MacDonald's conclusions are:

1. Tissue inflammation is not seen in fetuses with transplacentally-acquired infection with the Lyme spirochete.

2. Lyme disease acquired in utero may result in fetal death in utero, fetal death at term or infant death after birth. Babies may also survive in spite of the bacteria being isolated in the placenta.

3. In all but one of these cases where the Lyme organism was identified in the placenta or the fetal tissues, the maternal blood had no evidence of antibodies to the Lyme bacteria. In only two of the fourteen cases was there a maternal history compatible with Lyme disease, yet neither of the two were serologically confirmed.

This is the extent of the currently available information on Lyme and Pregnancy in the medical literature in 1990. Comparing the various studies have led us to arrive at the following conclusions:

1. Lyme disease is a serious threat to pregnant women in that it may cause fetal damage and death.

2. Pregnancy may mask symptoms of Lyme in the mother and may result in seronegativity.

3. Serologic screening of pregnant women in highly endemic areas is not recommended.

4. Pregnant women who test positive for Lyme antibodies, yet have no symptoms suggesting active Lyme, are probably at a lower risk of passing the infection across the placenta. It may be possible that the presence of antibody prevents the Borrelia burgdorferi from crossing the placenta.

5. Babies born with Lyme disease can be expected to have a negative blood test for Lyme antibodies. Few have positive tests.

6. We desperately need a better test for detecting Lyme in pregnant women. It is clear that serologies are inadequate.

> Efforts should be directed at evaluating urine antigen and PCR testing in pregnancy and in neonates.

In our practice we have seen several dozen pregnant women with Lyme disease. I feel that a much more aggressive approach must be taken with them than with non-pregnant patients. It is preferable to err on the side of overtreatment than under treatment, especially since the antibiotics we use have not been associated with birth defects or adverse effects on the developing fetus. These are general recommendations that we have developed over the last three years:

A pregnant woman who presents with a deer tick bite in an endemic area for Lyme disease is treated as if she had Stage 1 Lyme disease. We would treat with one to two months of oral antibiotics, such as Amoxicillin or Ceftin. (Tetracycline and Doxycycline are contraindicated in pregnancy.)

A pregnant woman with an EM rash should receive three to four weeks of intravenous Claforan, Rocephin or aqueous penicillin. We have evidence that even without constitutional symptoms the Lyme spirochete may have spread throughout the mother's body by the fifth day after an infected tick bite. As noted above, treatment failure with oral penicillin has been reported.

Pregnant women who are diagnosed as having Lyme by symptoms and blood tests, who do not have a clear history of a tick bite or EM rash, and have not yet been treated, should be treated with intravenous antibiotics. Here, since the length of infection is unknown, we must assume that the spirochetes have spread throughout the mother's body. It has generally been assumed that it is only possible to culture the Lyme spirochete from the blood only in the early stages of Lyme disease, so that a woman in the later stages of Lyme is safe from having blood-borne spirochetes reaching and crossing the placenta to the fetus. Yet unpublished data suggests that blood drawn from chronic Lyme patients during the afternoon, when they usually spike a mild fever, may yield spirochetes, using a specially modified BS Kelly culture Medium. Animal studies with chronically infected dogs show that when their immune systems are suppressed by injecting them with dexamethasone, a steroid similar to prednisone, it is possible to culture the Lyme spirochete from their blood the day after the injection. It may be possible that the state of pregnancy, which is also immunosuppressive, may induce the spirochete to enter the bloodstream and reach the placenta.

We recommend that pregnant women with active Lyme, or a history of treated Lyme, have monthly urine antigen tests for Lyme until the seventh month of pregnancy. There is some evidence that during the 3rd trimester, false positive urine tests may occur.

When the baby is delivered, we recommend that the placenta be examined for spirochetes. If spirochetes are demonstrated in the placenta, the baby should be treated with intravenous antibiotics.

I must again stress that these are guidelines that we use in our own practice. I realize that many physicians might criticize them for being an over-reaction and too aggressive: however, I have seen a number of babies born with congenital Lyme, and am quite aware of the devastating effects it can cause. Following the recommendations I've outlined above, we have had normal outcomes in all the pregnant women whom we have treated. **[End Article]**

RECENT STUDIES

Dr. John Drulle's research (presented above), although groundbreaking, was conducted several decades ago. Now we will examine recent scientific studies. The research substantiating Dr. Drulle's above article ended in 1990, so let's pick up the trail there.

The Department of Infectious Diseases, University Medical Centre, in Ljubljana, Slovenia examined the cases of 105 pregnant women (from 1990 to 1997) who presented during the course of their pregnancy with erythema migrans (erythema migrans is the scientific name for the telltale bulls-eye rash that positively identifies a Borrelia infection). The medical cases were tracked by the Lyme Borreliosis Outpatients' Clinic.[2] Nearly all of the affected women received aggressive antibiotic therapy, including benzyl penicillin (10 million IU b.i.d.) or ceftriaxone (2 g daily). 93 of 105 women delivered on time and had healthy babies. However, 12 babies (11.4%) experienced problems. Two pregnancies ended in involuntary abortion; six pregnancies ended with preterm birth; four babies were born with congenital anomalies; one baby was born with syndactyly; and three babies had urologic abnormalities that manifested by age 5. While the authors observe that "a causal association with borrelial infection was not proven," it is interesting to note that at least one of the preterm babies was born with a cardiac abnormality, one of the most common manifestations of Lyme disease.

In another study, *Przegl Epidemiol,* a Polish medical journal, reported in a 2004 issue the case of a 25-year-old woman living in an endemic area for Lyme disease who presented at a local hospital during her 29th week of pregnancy. Findings included thrombocytopenia, fever and fatigue. During the last few weeks of pregnancy, erythema migrans developed. The woman did not receive proper treatment. The infant was born with thrombocytopenia, and 3 months into life, developed erythema migrans.

---

[2] And you thought Lyme disease existed only in the United States! This "Lyme Borreliosis Outpatients' Clinic" is located in Slovenia. For more information on the prevalence of Lyme disease around the globe, read the *2008 Lyme disease Annual Report,* www.lymebook.com/lyme-annual-report.

The infant then tested positive for Lyme Borreliosis. According to the authors of this article, it was not positively confirmed that Lyme disease was transferred during pregnancy, however, the authors acknowledge that such transfer is a possibility.

A telling and eye-opening study conducted by The Department of Obstetrics and Gynecology, University of Alabama at Birmingham, and published in the September, 2003 issue of *American Journal of Obstetrics and Gynecology* set out to "determine the relationship between various types of perinatal infections and stillbirths." The authors of the study reviewed various textbooks and surveyed MEDLINE articles. In a concluding paragraph of the study, the authors write:

> *"Infection may cause stillbirth by a number of mechanisms, including direct infection, placental damage, and severe maternal illness. A large variety of organisms have been associated with stillbirth, including many bacteria, viruses, and protozoa...leptospirosis, Q fever, and Lyme disease have all been implicated as etiologic for stillbirth."*

The important implications of this study are three-fold: First, not only can maternal infections have a significant effect on unborn children; they can actually lead to stillbirth. Second, Lyme disease is not the only microorganism implicated in fetal damage—viruses, bacteria, and protozoa may also be involved. Third, severe maternal illness has been found to accompany the subsequent placental damage—keep this in mind when you read the mothers' stories in Appendix E.

In addition to screening mothers and children for Lyme disease, it is also telling to look for the infection in the placentas of women who are known to be infected. After all, the placenta is responsible for nurturing the fetus, and should the placenta become infected, it would follow that a higher risk exists for fetal infection. In 1996, The Department of Obstetrics and Gynecology at New York Medical College in the Westchester County Medical

Center undertook such a study and found that 5% of 60 mothers who tested positive for Borrelia infection had placentas which also tested positive for the infection. While 5% is a relatively low number, it is necessary to keep in mind the possibility of false negative test results in the 95% which had placentas that tested negative. Additionally, the women chosen for the study were asymptomatic even though they tested positive for Borrelia. It is possible that women with more severe infections and/or symptoms may be harboring more bacteria, and hence, a higher probability of an infected placenta.

One of the most profound and influential studies was conducted in 1995 by the Department of Obstetrics and Gynecology, University of Utah School of Medicine, Salt Lake City. This study looked at the outcome of pregnancy in infected mice, and the results are shocking. Fetal death occurred in 33 of 280 pregnancies among infected mice, while uninfected control mice experienced 0 fetal deaths in 191 pregnancies. PCR testing found Borrelia DNA in the uteri of some infected mice, and spirochete DNA was present in several tissue samples taken from fetuses of infected mice. Interestingly, the study found that acute Borrelia infection was more dangerous than chronic Borrelia infection in terms of fetus outcome. This single study, without the support of the other studies presented in this book, offers a strong case for the potential for Lyme disease to be transferred during pregnancy.

In another study, chronic Lyme disease was implied to be more dangerous than acute Lyme disease, in contrast to the above study. The Department of Pediatrics at New York Medical College published in 1993 the results of their review of over two thousand cases of prenatal exposure to Lyme disease. Approximately 2000 Westchester County, New York women completed questionnaires and had sera tested for antibodies to Borrelia burgdorferi at their first prenatal visit and again at delivery. Researchers found that while tick bites that occurred around the time of conception had little or no negative impact on the babies, "tick bites within 3 years preceding conception were significantly associated with congenital malformations." This implies that the longer the infection has been present in the mother's body, the more likely it will be that adverse fetal effects occur.

Lyme-infected dogs were studied by the University of Wisconsin School of Veterinary Medicine, and results were published in a 1993 article, the purpose of which was to examine "whether or not intra-uterine transmission of Borrelia burgdorferi could exist in dogs." Ten female Beagles were inoculated intradermally with approximately 1,000 Borrelia organisms; inoculation was repeated every two weeks during the gestation period. Ten control Beagles were inoculated on a similar schedule with placebo saline solution. The dogs were then bred naturally; both control and infected groups. Blood from the puppies was collected on day one of life and then subsequently each week until six weeks old. An astounding 80% of infected mothers gave birth to litters that had at least one infected puppy. In several litters, in addition to positive PCR test results, the physical presence of spirochetes was actually detected, confirming the existence of the infection. This is another study which, if standing alone (irrespective of the other supporting studies presented in this chapter), would be sufficient evidence for building a strong argument for transplacental transfer of Lyme disease. A similar animal study conducted by the same school of veterinary medicine, published a few months later, found that Lyme disease can be transferred through the placenta in cows as well.

When considering whether or not Lyme disease may be transmitted during pregnancy, it is helpful to look at Lyme's cousin, Syphilis. Lyme disease and Syphilis are both spirochetal diseases and share many characteristics. In terms of neurological involvement, Syphilis is associated primarily with derangement of grey matter in the brain, while Lyme disease is associated primarily with derangement of white matter in the brain. Also, Syphilis is known to be congenitally transferred, hence, it is logical to conclude that Lyme disease may also be congenitally transferred. When discussing Syphilis, congenital transfer is not theory or speculation; it is proven, accepted fact. According to the United States Centers for Disease Control informational website on Syphilis (CDC):

> *Effective prevention and detection of congenital Syphilis depends on the identification of Syphilis in pregnant women and, therefore, on the routine serologic screening of pregnant women during the first prenatal visit. In communities and populations in which the risk for congenital Syphilis is high, serologic testing and a sexual history also should be obtained at 28 weeks' gestation and at delivery...No infant or mother should leave the hospital unless the maternal serologic status has been documented at least once during pregnancy, and at delivery in communities and populations in which the risk for congenital Syphilis is high.*

If it is accepted science that Syphilis can be sexually and congenitally transferred, then why not Lyme disease, as well? Are not Syphilis and Lyme disease highly similar spirochetal infections? Consider the evidence and decide for yourself.

Family Disease Trends

If Lyme disease can be passed down through families via transfer during pregnancy, then you would expect to see symptoms of Lyme disease in mothers who give birth to autistic children and, perhaps, entire families—maybe even extended families. People in these families would have a two-fold risk for contracting Lyme disease (and/or autism): First, they would be at risk for contracting one or both of these disorders from a tick bite—both Lyme disease and autism are most prevalent in areas where ticks thrive, and where ticks are likely to carry Lyme disease (see Chapter 6). Second, they would be at risk of transfer during the gestation phase of life, due to parental transfer.

And this is precisely what we observe. Tami Duncan is in contact with hundreds of mothers with autistic children. Most such mothers in the United States do not know about the Lyme-autism connection, however, when they are alerted to the connection (either by the efforts of Tami through the LIA Foundation or other research avenues), they quickly become keenly aware of the strange illnesses riddling family members who have a direct blood relationship with the autistic children in the family. Typical illnesses observed among family members are, astoundingly, those which are intimately tied to Lyme disease, including chronic fatigue syndrome, fibromyalgia, and a slew of mental disorders. Appendix E includes some of these families' stories.

The amount of published research on the topic of familial disease clustering is staggering, and numerous books would need to be written to accommodate all of the available science. In this section, instead of unabridged coverage, we will instead present highlights of some key, relevant research.

The most important published study on family disease as it relates to autism was released in 1999 in the *Journal of Child Neurology*. Entitled "Familial Clustering of Autoimmune Disorders and Evaluation of Medical Risk Factors in Autism," the study was authored by Anne M. Comi, MD, Andrew W. Zimmerman, MD, Virginia H. Frye, EdD, Paul A. Law, MD, MPH, and Joseph N. Peeden, MD. The study set out to determine whether or not there is a correlation between autism and family disease, specifically autoimmune disease.[3]

---

[3] Current research is increasingly finding infectious etiology in autoimmune diseases. Once believed to be caused exclusively by the body's unwarranted attack on itself, autoimmune disease is now widely believed to instead be caused by the body's warranted, yet misguided, attack on some type of stealth bacterial, viral, or fungal infection—and in some cases, that infection may be Lyme disease itself.

The study surveyed the families of 61 autistic patients and 46 healthy control subjects using questionnaires. The study found that "the mean number of autoimmune disorders was greater in families with autism; 46% had two or more members with autoimmune disorders...As the number of family members with autoimmune disorders increased from one to three, the risk of autism was greater." These findings are precisely consistent with the hypothesis that autism is both transferable within families and of an infectious etiology. Additionally, the study found that of sick family members, the highest correlation to autistic children was sick mothers, further confirming the possibility of transfer between mother and child. While both mother and father pass on their genetics to the child, only the mother has the intimate contact with the baby necessary to pass on an infection.

Furthermore, the specific autoimmune disorders discovered in some families of autistic children have long been suspected to be Lyme disease "in disguise." These include type 1 diabetes, adult rheumatoid arthritis, hypothyroidism, and systemic lupus erythematosus. Seizures were also present in some families.

Anyone with even a cursory Lyme disease education knows that arthritis is one of the primary symptoms of Lyme disease, and that people diagnosed with rheumatoid arthritis are often really suffering from Lyme disease. The connection between Lupus and Lyme disease is not as obvious; however, it is indeed a reality—as illustrated by lupus patients who improve on the Marshall Protocol, a protocol which was developed to treat infectious bacteria including Borrelia burgdorferi. Seizures, of course, are also one of the primary symptoms of Lyme disease. The study concludes by stating that, "An increased number of autoimmune disorders suggests that in some families with autism, immune dysfunction could interact with various environmental factors to play a role in autism pathogenesis."

A study released just prior to this book's publication, on May 5, 2008, found that mothers (but not fathers) with schizophrenia, personality disorders, or depression were twice as likely as healthy mothers to give birth to autistic children. The study was conducted in Sweden and was made possible by the nation's detailed national health registry which renders statistical data easy to access and analyze. Again, interestingly, a father's mental illness did not appear to be a factor in having an autistic child. Also of note was the fact that drug addiction and alcohol in either parent was not a risk factor for autism (eliminating yet another possible causative variable). Schizophrenia, personality disorders, and depression are disorders which can be mimicked by an underlying Lyme infection.

Additional studies reveal even more piercing insights. Recently, in 2005, the *Journal of Autism and Developmental Disorders* published a study co-sponsored by the Division of Pediatric Neurology, Duke University, and the Department of Neurology, Tufts New England Medical Center. This study found that autism is more likely to occur in families with a history of bipolar disorder. Lyme disease is primarily a neurological disorder, and bipolar disorder is one of the most well-known and insidious of neurological Lyme disease symptoms. Autism and bipolar disorder are completely different diseases, with completely different symptoms and courses. Yet, the two diseases are linked within families. Why such an unlikely pair? The Lyme-autism connection is a hypothesis that offers a workable explanation: as we have seen, Lyme disease can be transferred from mother to child during pregnancy, which explains the inter-family connection, and Lyme disease manifests in a broad range of neurological symptom pictures, which explains the connection between autism and bipolar disorder, two seemingly unrelated mental health disorders.

The Division of Pediatric Neurology also published findings in 1994 similar to those described in the above 2005 report. In 1994, it was found that "...an important subgroup of autistic spectrum disorders may be related etiologically to familial major affective disorders, and may represent the early-life onset of a severe phenotype of major affective, particularly bipolar, disease."

In London, similar conclusions are being reached. The Genetic and Developmental Psychiatry Research Centre published in 1998 a study entitled "Autism, affective and other psychiatric disorders: patterns of familial aggregation." The report was released by Cambridge University Press in the Journal of Psychological Medicine. Researchers found that "Motor tics, obsessive–compulsive disorder (OCD) and affective disorders were significantly more common in relatives of autistic probands... Direct interview data confirmed the increased rate of affective disorders (especially major depressive disorder) in the first-degree relatives." Obsessive compulsive disorder? Motor tics? Affective disorder and depression? These are *hallmark symptoms* of Lyme disease. Are these findings in family members mere coincidence?

Maybe it was just the stress of raising an autistic child that induced these mental disorders in first-degree relatives. No—the London researchers denounced the possibility that parental mental disorders were caused by the stress of raising developmentally challenged children: "The increased risk of affective disorders was not solely the consequence of the stress of raising a child with autism and further research will be required to clarify the mechanisms involved."

What about other childhood developmental disorders? Do they also have family roots? In a study conducted by the University of Iowa College of Medicine, it was found that parents of autistic children scored considerably worse than parents of children with

Down syndrome, on tests of intelligence, reading and spelling, IQ, and executive function.

Interpreting the Data and Moving Past the Genetics Paradigm

So what does all of this data mean? In this chapter we have seen that Lyme disease can be transferred from mother to child during pregnancy. We also described how the diseases which are mimicked by Lyme disease are common in the immediate families of autistic children. If we put 2 and 2 together—congenital transfer and family groupings—we end up with the strong probability that not only can Lyme disease be transferred to an unborn baby, but also that the acquired infection can cause autism and/or similar mental disorders.

Additionally, we can refute the common assertion that heredity is the only factor to be blamed for diseases passed down in families. Although genetics are to be blamed sometimes, stealth bacterial infections such as Lyme disease have not received due consideration in the process of passing disease down through families. It is time for researchers to give the same attention to infections as they give to genes and genetics.

Although slow, researchers are beginning to make this journey and look into non-genetic factors in familial disease. For example, Susan L. Smalley, Ph.D., James McCracken, and Peter Tanguay of the Department of Psychiatry, University of California, Los Angeles, recently published a study entitled "Autism, affective disorders, and social phobia," in which they set out to "test the hypothesis that major affective and/or anxiety disorders are increased among relatives of autistic probands compared with controls." The results indicated that non-genetic familial disorders, including major depressive disorder and social phobia, had a much higher correlation with autism than did genetic disorders. Given the context of our present discussion, these findings are not surprising, as the condition which facilitates transfer of Lyme disease during pregnancy is not genetic, but instead, completely circumstantial. It is as simple as asking the question, "Does the mom have Lyme disease and if so, did she pass it down to her child or children?" No genetics involved, but instead, only the simple passing of living bacteria from one human to another. The lack of a genetic component is profound and should not be overlooked. If not genetics, then what? A transferrable bacterial infection fits the bill.

Also of note in the above study is the shocking finding that, again, the familial disorders which precede autism in the family tree are in fact the same disorders which Lyme disease mimics, e.g., social phobia, affective disorders, and depression.

Refuting the Inevitable Guilt

All this talk of familial background might make you start to feel guilty. Is it your fault that your child has autism? Of course not—no more than it is to your credit that your child might have above average athletic abilities. The fact that you are reading this book demonstrates that your intention is to become as educated as possible in order to give your child the greatest chance of a full recovery. You should feel the opposite of guilt. You should feel proud of yourself for stepping up to the plate and doing all you can. Your research and dedication offers your child a better chance at life.

In fact, the perpetuation of Lyme-autism research holds nothing but hope and a brighter future for kids. If Lyme disease does cause, or at least, contribute to, the onset of autism, then proper Lyme disease screening, diagnosis, and treatment in women of reproductive age could prevent some cases of autism. In the words of Tami Duncan, published in *The Townsend Letter for Doctors and Patients*[4],

> *"...there is a desperate need for an autism prevention program. Testing young women for these infections before they conceive is imperative and providing proper treatment to minimize transmission to the fetus is essential. What if half of the autism cases could be prevented? ... The Lyme-autism connection currently appears to affect 20-30% of children with autism spectrum disorder. This is a large subset and can potentially be prevented if young mothers are educated on proper health, testing for heavy metals and infections prior to conceiving. I am interested in communicating with physicians who would like to assist in creating an autism prevention program."*

Any guilt or feelings of self-condemnation should be replaced by hope, a vigorous desire to keep researching, and the recognition that you have done, and are doing, everything in your power to be a loving parent.

At this point in the book, completing Chapter 2, many questions remained unanswered and the foundation for the Lyme-autism connection still requires some additional substantiation. Now that we have presented evidence which establishes the plausibility of congenital transfer of the Borrelia infection, and the likelihood that such an infection can lead to autism, let's move on to the next piece of the puzzle addressed in Chapter 3: the autis-

---

[4] The Townsend Letter for Doctors and Patients is a monthly periodical whose vision is to be the "Examiner of Alternative Medicine." This periodical is one of the most valuable sources for updated information on cutting-edge Lyme disease and autism research. With a circulation of approximately 10,000, the journal is read by the leading minds of alternative medicine in America. Not just for physicians, the publication is also targeted to patients. Tami Duncan, co-founder of the LIA Foundation, is a regular contributing writer for The Townsend Letter For Doctors and Patients, as are numerous other physicians and researchers at the centers of the fields of Lyme disease and autism research. In addition to signing up for a regular subscription, you would also benefit from special-ordering the April, 2007 issue, which focused on Lyme disease and included numerous useful articles on all kinds of conventional and alternative treatments. The Lyme-autism connection is mentioned often in this periodical.

tic child's immune system. After exploring this topic, Chapter 3 will also look at scientific studies examining infectious involvement in autism. Later in the book, additional chapters will con-continue to add pieces to the puzzle by addressing symptomology, geographic incidence, and an in-depth Lyme-autism study.

Chapter 3
Immunity and Infections in Autism

Building the Case

In building the case for the Lyme-autism connection, the next step in the journey is to determine whether or not autism involves immune system irregularities. In the previous chapter we explored the possibility that Lyme disease may potentially be transferred from mother to child during pregnancy. However, if autism does not involve the immune system, then we would be hard-pressed to implicate Lyme disease (an infection that causes immune system activity) as a causative factor in autism. In other words, in order for the Lyme-autism connection to be possible, it must first be shown that autistic pathology involves the type of immune function and dysfunction also seen in Lyme disease.

The primary function of the human immune system is to fight infections. So, if a particular disease results in changes to the immune system, it can be reasonably concluded that infections play a role in that disease process.

What do we find when looking at autism? We find that immune system changes, malfunction, and radical abnormalities exist in autistic children. Understanding these immune system irregularities is the first step to laying the foundation for understanding the role infections (and Lyme disease) play in autism. Let's take a brief tour through some of the relevant science.

In October of 1998, Michigan's College of Pharmacy reported in the Journal of Clinical Immunology and Immunopathology that antibodies found in the blood of autistic children suggest that the brain dysfunction in autism may be the result of autoimmune response to exposure to viruses and mycoplasma bacteria. Joseph Mercola, DO, one of the most respected alternative physicians in the United States, responded to this finding with the following comment:

> *"One possibility is that early exposure to a virus prods the body into mounting an immune response that somehow goes awry. In addition to producing antibodies against the virus, the body makes antibodies against itself, resulting in damage to tissues and organs."*

Johns Hopkins discovered a similar phenomenon and published a fascinating study in the Annals of Neurology on November 15, 2004. This was one of the groundbreaking studies that revealed clear signs of inflammation in the brains of autistic children. According to Carlos Pardo-Villamizar, MD, assistant professor of neurology and pathology at Johns Hopkins and senior author of the study, "These findings reinforce the theory that immune response in the brain is involved in autism, although it is not yet clear whether the inflammation is a consequence of disease or a cause of it, or both."

Pardo-Villamizar goes on to comment that the study focused specifically on the levels of cytokines and chemokines found in the cerebrospinal fluid of autistic patients ranging in age from 5 to 12 years old. When compared with normal controls, the brains and spinal fluid of autistic people were found to have ongoing inflammatory processes. Additionally, after conducting tissue samples, researchers found that specific regions of the brain seemed to be more affected.

It seems likely that these regions may be victim of some type of infection that is the root cause of the inflammation. Pardo-Villamizar acknowledges this possibility in one of the concluding statements of the study: "These findings suggest that the inflammation is localized to specific regions within the brain and not caused by immune system abnormalities from outside the brain." What a telling statement! Whereas other types of immune system dysfunction may result from non-specific, generalized abnormalities in the body, this statement implies that inflammation in the autistic brain is localized, specific, and isolated. This conclusion is compatible with the hypothesis that neurological infections, and Lyme disease in particular, have causative activity in autism. Lyme disease is known to infect and cause inflammation in specific regions in the brain.

You can add UC Davis to the list of research organizations that have discovered immune system abnormalities in autistic children. In 2005, a study conducted by M.I.N.D. Institute and the NIEHS Center for Children's Environmental Health illustrated that autistic children respond to bacterial and viral challenges differently than healthy children. Specifically, researchers discovered that the activity of various immune system cells, including B cells and T cells, as well as response by cytokine, an immune system protein, were deranged in autistic immune systems after challenge by bacterial and viral infections.

Among the other interesting findings of this study was the statistic that autism now affects one in every 166 children. Again, a disease with skyrocketing incidence, similar to Lyme disease, whose numbers are also showing explosive growth.

Researchers found that autistic children sometimes feel better when they have a fever. Martha Herbert, an assistant professor in neurology at the Harvard Medical School and research advisor for the Autism Society of America, hypothesizes that one of the reasons for this may be increased activity of cytokines, which are immune cells active in the presence of infection. This study was published in the Journal of Pediatrics.

One of the most significant indicators that autism is a disorder related to immune function was discovered in a study conducted by the Division of Basic and Clinical Immunology, University of California, Irvine. This study was published in the *Journal of Autism and Developmental Disorders* in August of 1996. Entitled "Dysregulated immune system in children with autism: beneficial effects of intravenous immune globulin on autistic characteristics," this study found (as the title implies) that IV immune globulin actually helped the symptoms of autism in a number of children. This is a profound discovery because, if autism were unrelated to the immune system, then such treatment should be completely benign and have no effects, positive or negative. Additionally, it is interesting to note that one of the most helpful treatments in reducing symptoms of patients with confirmed Lyme disease is, you guessed it, IV immune globulin treatment.

An earlier study (1986, Primary Children's Medical Center, Salt Lake City, UT) also published in the *Journal of Autism and Developmental Disorders* described similar findings, although this time, instead of measuring response to treatment with immune globulin, the study simply took blood measurements of various immune markers. The summary of the study speaks for itself:

> *We have begun an investigation on the immune systems of patients with autism in attempt to determine if immune mechanisms are*

involved in the development of this severe developmental disorder. A study of 31 autistic patients has revealed several immune-system abnormalities, including reduced responsiveness in the lymphocyte blastogenesis assay to phytohemagglutinin, concanavalin A, and pokeweed mitogen; decreased numbers of T lymphocytes; and an altered ratio of helper to suppressor T cells. Immune-system abnormalities may be directly related to underlying biologic processes of autism, or these changes may be an indirect reflection of the actual pathologic mechanism.

Note that several of these abnormal findings are also present in many Lyme disease patients, including, of particular note, altered ratio of helper to suppressor T cells and decreased numbers of T lymphocytes.

What is so significant about the differences between the autistic immune system and a healthy person's immune system? There are several important implications, the Lyme-autism connection itself being only one.

First, these differences show that autism is physiological in nature, and that the common behavioral therapies often used to treat autism, while helpful, will not address the underlying physiological problems. In the words of UC Davis, "...autism, currently defined primarily by distinct behaviors, may potentially be defined by distinct biologic changes as well...understanding the biology of autism is crucial to developing better ways to diagnose and treat it." Autism is a physical disease, not a psychiatric disorder.

Second, the autistic immune system is screaming at the top of its lungs to researchers, saying "please investigate infection as a possible cause of my plight—I am sounding all the alarms of invasion by foreign microorganisms!"

Third, the characteristics of the autistic immune system which we have just examined serve to set the stage for the next subjects we will discuss: the science supporting the role of infections in the pathology of autism, and finally, the science that supports Lyme disease in the pathology of autism.

Autism and Infections

Having seen that it is possible for Lyme disease to be transferred during pregnancy, and that autism involves immune system dysfunction / activation, we can now move on to look specifically at the presence of various infections in autism. This is one more element in setting the stage for the Lyme-autism connection. We introduced this topic in the introduction of the book, and now we will take a more in-depth look at some of the science.

Garth Nicolson, Ph.D., president and founder of *The Institute for Molecular Medicine,* www.immed.org, has the following to say about the role of infections in autism. This excerpt was taken from a journal article published in 2007 in the *Infectious Disease Newsletter.*

> *"Patients with neurodegenerative and behavioral disorders often have systemic bacterial, viral and/or fungal infections that may play important roles in their pathogenesis…we have examined patients with ALS, Multiple Sclerosis, and autism-spectrum disorders (including autism, attention deficit disorder, and Asperger's Syndrome) and found evidence for systemic intracellular bacterial and viral infections in the majority of patients."*

Figure 2 (next page), from *The Institute for Molecular Medicine,* indicates that laboratory testing not only found Borrelia to be present in autistic children, but also several other infections.

The topic of autism and infections is a massive one, and dozens of pages have been written and published over the past several decades. This book will by no means attempt to rewrite literature that is already available. Instead, we will take only a cursory look at the topic, saving the majority of our focus for the Lyme-autism connection. The topic of general infections as they relate to autism is relevant here because it bridges the gap between the broad immune system dysfunction in autism and the specific relationship between Lyme disease and autism.

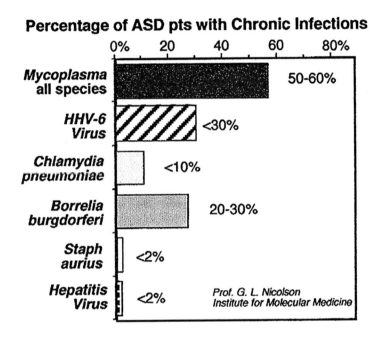

Percent incidence of bacterial and viral infections in 48 patients with Autistic Spectrum Disorders (ASD). The range indicates results from different laboratories.

FIGURE 2

To understand the connection between autism and infections, you must first understand some basic concepts relating to the brain. When we talk about other organs, such as the stomach, heart, or lungs, everyone knows that problems with these organs result from physical disturbances in their function. No one thinks to him or herself, "my asthma must be caused by my personality," or, "that heart attack I had was a result of bad parenting when I was a child." These are silly assertions. While psychological well-being definitely can affect the physical function of organs, we all know that dysfunction in organs is a result of something that is physically wrong with those organs.

The same realization must be applied when thinking about brain dysfunction. The discipline of psychiatry has led to numerous false conclusions about the brain. Psychiatrists often talk about emotional, behavioral, and experiential factors as precipitating forces in the onset of mental illness. While this can be true in some cases, many instances of mental illness are a direct result of physical assaults against the brain which have nothing to do with psychological factors. Consider the famous example that appears in college neurology textbooks describing a normal person who ends up, as the result of a work accident, with a 6-inch railroad nail penetrating and becoming lodged in the frontal lobe of his brain. The person experienced numerous psychiatric symptoms which could have otherwise been blamed on his upbringing, the parenting he received, or other experiential factors. The fascinating part of this example is that some of the changes noted were subtle personality nuances which would have previously, according to science, been attributed to nothing more than social and cultural influence. The example of the railroad nail incident shows that a physical insult to the brain can lead to behavioral and psychiatric manifestations. Use of recreational drugs is another example—physical substances which have very real behavioral and psychological consequences.

And so it is with neurological infections. Similar to a 6-inch nail becoming lodged in your brain, neurological infections are a direct trauma to the brain. Bacteria, fungi, and viruses that establish infection in the brain cause physical trauma to brain tissue and result in the same type of psychological disturbances that would occur if you had been hit on the head with a rock or had a 6-inch nail thrust into your skull. Just as suffering from strep throat (a bacterial infection) can cause your throat to become red and inflamed, so infections of the brain can cause brain function to become compromised.

One doctor who understands this principle is Dr. Robert Bransfield. "Lyme disease is like an injury of the brain," he says. If you get time, don't miss his groundbreaking article entitled *Microbes and Mental Illness*, accessible by pointing your browser to:

www.mentalhealthandillness.com/Articles/MicrobesAndMentalIllness.htm

There are numerous other interesting articles available on his website. As you read the rest of this book, keep in mind the very real, physical nature of neurological infections.

A Few Example Infections

A complete list of the various infections involved in autism is beyond the scope of this book. Many books and articles have already been written on the topic. In the next page or two, however, we will look at a few examples of infections which are known with certainty to be involved in autism. The goal here is to build a bridge toward the Lyme-autism connection. If we know that numerous other infections are involved in autism, it is a shorter leap to make to conclude that Lyme disease may also be involved.

In 2003, one of the most important and influential autism textbooks was published. Entitled *Autism Spectrum Disorders*, and edited by Eric Hollander, this book broke open the topic of infections as potential causative factors in autism, and listed dozens of potential infective agents, along with the published scientific studies supporting infection in autism. The following are some of the infectious agents proven to be associated with the onset of autism:

Rubella. Prenatal rubella infection in the mother was found to be associated with autism when children contracted rubella in utero, according to a study that analyzed the 1964 rubella epidemic in New York City. Interestingly, Hollander notes that Rubella-induced autism is accompanied by symptoms that differ from autism induced by other causes.

Human Herpesvirus-6. This infection has been identified in autistic children by antibody-positive sera, and a strong correlation has been observed between children who test positive for this antibody and children who develop autism.

Herpes Simplex. Numerous studies have connected herpes simplex encephalitis with autism. Of particular note is the case of an 11-year-old girl who, after a bout with acute encephalopathic illness, developed full-blown autism. Test results showed brain lesions in the temporal lobe region. The temporal lobe region of the brain is not only the region affected by herpes simplex encephalopathy, but is also believed to be the region affected by autism. Other studies identified children who experienced similar late-onset autism after exposure to the herpes virus. Amazingly, some of the autistic-like syndromes that developed were fully reversible (possibly because they were acquired later in life).

Measles. According to Hollander, *"a study on the association of various prenatal and early postnatal viral exposures with autism found an association between prenatal measles (i.e., maternal measles infection) and autism."* It should come as no surprise that measles virus might induce a neurological disorder such as autism (especially when the exposure occurs at a young and tender age). Even adult cases of measles have been associated with neurological sequelae.

Stealth Viruses. Far ahead of its time, this autism book has actually acknowledged the existence of stealth viruses which have not yet been identified by modern medicine, and further-more, the book notes that such viruses may play a causative role in the development of autism.

Interestingly, even the flu virus can increase the risk of autism, according to Utah State University. In a study published in the *Journal of Neuroscience*, in January, 2003, Utah State Universi-ty reports that,

> *Maternal viral infection is known to increase the risk for schizophrenia and autism in the offspring. Using this observation in an animal model, we find that respiratory infection of pregnant mice with the human influenza virus yields offspring that display highly abnormal behavioral responses as adults. As in schizophrenia and autism, these offspring display deficits in prepulse inhibition (PPI) in the acoustic startle response. Compared with control mice, the infected mice also display striking responses to the acute administration of antipsychotic (clozapine and chlorpromazine) and psychomimetic (ketamine) drugs. Moreover, these mice are deficient in exploratory behavior in both open-field and novel-object tests, and they are deficient in social interaction.*

University of California, Irvine researchers conducted an intri-guing study entitled *An infection-based model of neuro-developmental damage.* In this study, it was found that "peri-natal exposure to infectious agents and toxins is linked to the pathogenesis of psychiatric disorders." The study involved inocu-lating rats intracerebrally with various infectious microorganisms. It was found that behavior among infected rats resembled autism. Specifically, the study found "abnormalities of hippocampal and cerebellar development, growth, play behavior, and learning that correlate with disturbances observed in some children with autism." Furthermore, infected rats displayed changes in cytokine function, an immune cell that is often present during infection.

After looking at the above research, and noting the many infec-tious agents that can contribute to autism, it may seem that the

Lyme-autism connection is less likely because, presumably, almost any infection can cause (or contribute to) autism. You may be asking, then, why we have chosen to single out Lyme disease as a key infection. Why not write a book on the Rubella-autism connection? Or how about the Herpes-autism connection? The answer to this question might surprise you. We can easily concede that a Rubella-autism connection or a Herpes-autism connection is just as likely (or nearly as likely) as a Lyme-autism connection. In fact, some cases of autism are probably caused by those and other microorganisms.

So why the book you now hold in your hands? Why focus specifically on the Lyme disease infection? The answer to this question is simple. Of all the infections which could potentially be involved in autism, Lyme disease is one of the only modern infections undergoing a rapid increase in incidence, following roughly the same curve as the radically increasing incidence of autism. If the primary infectious agent in autism were Rubella, how would we explain why autism cases are climbing at an explosive rate, while the rate of Rubella cases is nearly insignificant? This is yet another piece of the Lyme-autism puzzle which, when set on the table, takes its place in the big picture. See Chapter 6 for an in-depth statistical analysis of the paralleling incidences of Lyme disease and autism.

By this point in the book, we have looked at numerous scientific studies surrounding Lyme disease and autism, but no studies that look specifically at the Lyme-autism connection itself. As noted in the introduction, it was necessary to build the majority of our argument in this fashion since direct studies are few and far between. Having now built the foundation established in the first half of the book, let's turn our attention to one of the only available studies that focuses specifically on the Lyme-autism connection. This study is the focus of Chapter 4.

Chapter 4
Making the Connection

In this chapter, we will begin by looking at several clues which can be seen when autism is treated with antibiotics, and we will then examine the key scientific study that supports the Lyme-autism connection hypothesis. We will also look at several supporting studies, and discuss some of the studies which are currently (at the time this book was written) in-progress.

The Antibiotic Clue

Although the official theory about the connection between Lyme disease and autism is fairly new, as is the organization that was established to study the link (the LIA Foundation), researchers have been noticing clues in this direction for years. Take, for example, unofficial research conducted in 2000 in which Dr. Richard Sandler of Rush Children's Hospital, Chicago, Illinois, treated 11 autistic children with the antibiotic vancomycin. Because the treatment of choice for Lyme disease is also antibiotics (Lyme disease is a bacterial infection), this study was interesting—even though Dr. Sandler did not specifically consider Lyme disease as a factor in the research.

According to the Associated Press, the story began when an Illinois mother, Ellen Bolte, "persuaded scientists to try a bizarre-sounding experiment, testing whether vancomycin might help her son's severe autism, which involved painful gastrointestinal symptoms which she hypothesized to be bacterial in nature. To their surprise, little Andrew Bolte got better." The article goes on:

> *"Dr. Richard Sandler of Rush Children's Hospital in Chicago was skeptical of Ellen's theory that a neurotoxin-producing intestinal infection was behind some of her son's symptoms. He administered the antibiotic anyway. Andrew 'was not cured, but all of a sudden he started saying words, and became toilet-trained,' Sandler recalled. 'I found that very intriguing. It's not supposed to happen.'"*

Subsequently, Sandler treated 11 other autistic children who also (similar to about a third of all autistic children) experienced painful gastrointestinal problems. After treatment, neuropsychological testing found that 10 of the 11 children improved. Results were reported in the Journal of Child Neurology.

Unfortunately, just a few months after the antibiotics were discontinued, Andrew and the others worsened again. Further study was postponed due to fears of overusing vancomycin, which could potentially lead to unwanted drug side effects as well as antibiotic-resistant bacterial outbreaks.

Although far from conclusive, the above unofficial study offers some important clues. First, antibiotics may have a positive effect in autism. This opens the door to the possibility that bacterial infections may play a role in autism. Second, the children deteriorated after the antibiotics were discontinued. This deterioration is a hallmark characteristic of chronic Lyme disease—many chronic Lyme patients take antibiotics on and off for years, finding that between courses of drugs, their symptoms return. This scenario is known as "relapsing and remitting chronic Lyme disease."

What of Ellen Bolte's hypothesis that the bacterial infection in question was located in her son's gastrointestinal tract? Is this hypothesis compatible with the Lyme-autism hypothesis?

Yes. Lyme disease does in fact colonize the intestinal tract, often leading to severe gastrointestinal symptoms. "So what," you may be thinking. "There are hundreds of other bacterial species which also have an effect on the intestinal tract—what foundation is there to blindly assume that the infection in question is Lyme disease instead of one of the many others? Is not such an assumption guilty of the logical fallacy known as 'begging the question'?"

Assuming Lyme disease is the true culprit would, in fact, be begging the question were it not for the other variables involved. The primary variable of interest is the fact that the vancomycin treatment did not just alleviate the intestinal problems, but also numerous neurological symptoms. While there are hundreds of potentially pathogenic bacterial strains that can colonize the digestive tract, few of them cause neurological symptoms. And fewer still cause neurological symptoms that are similar to those caused by Lyme disease. So, we can logically eliminate most pathogenic gastrointestinal bacterial strains from the list of possible offenders.

Take, for example, Clostridium difficile, also known as C. difficile, which is a very serious bacterial infection that can cause problems in the gastrointestinal tract. While this bacterial infection might seem suspect, it can be eliminated from the running due to the fact that it is not associated with neurological symptoms—instead, C. difficile is limited to causing such symptoms as watery diarrhea, fever, loss of appetite, nausea, and abdominal pain/tenderness. Are these symptoms those of neurological autism? No. Similarly, many other pathogenic bacteria can also be eliminated from the list of possible offenders for the same reason.

Interestingly, many parents and physicians have also noticed that antibiotic treatment can make autistic children worse, not better. At first glance, this observation may seem to cancel out the idea that antibiotic therapy can help autistic children improve. Or, the observation may lead to frustration, confusion, and a seemingly meaningless, contradictory data set. Yet, when this observation is viewed through the hypothetical lens of the Lyme-autism connection, the data is not contradictory or confusing, but instead very consistent and telling.

How can this be? Lyme disease is one of only a few bacterial infections which, when treated with antibiotics, leads to a reaction known as the Jarisch-Herxheimer reaction. This reaction is also sometimes referred to as a "herx," or "getting worse before you get better," or a "healing crisis." The herx reaction is documented to take place in Syphilis, Lyme disease, and a few other spirochetal illnesses. The reaction is named after two scientists who discovered the phenomenon. Adolf Jarisch (1850-1902), was an Austrian dermatologist who published his description of the reaction in 1895. Karl Herxheimer (1861-1944) was a German dermatologist who published his description of the reaction in 1902.

The definition of a herx reaction is an increase in the symptoms of a spirochetal disease (such as Syphilis, Lyme disease, or relapsing fever) occurring in some persons when treatment with spirocheticidal therapy is started. In the case of Lyme disease the herx reaction is an increase in the symptoms caused by neurotoxin circulation and inflammation.

1. **Increased neurotoxin circulation**. During normal lifecycle activities, the bacteria secretes neurotoxins. However, when

the spirochete is killed, an intense release of neurotoxins from dying bacterial organisms floods the body. Increased neurotoxin circulation can last from a few hours to a few weeks, depending on the sufficiency of a person's detoxification pathways as well as the extent of the kill-off.

2. **Increased inflammation.** When treating a spirochetal infection with antibiotics, an inflammatory response will result as the immune system is activated by the circulating antigens (protein codes which alert the immune system to the presence of an invader) released by dying bacterial organisms.

The herx reaction can vary from person to person, depending on the extent of the infection, location of infected areas, and body constitution. After the herx reaction has subsided, improvement is generally seen because the "bacterial load" (a term used to quantify the number of bacterial organisms in the body) has decreased due to the treatment.

Thus, the seeming paradox of antibiotic therapy leading to both improvement and worsening in autistic children is not a paradox at all when understood in the context of the Lyme-autism connection. Worsening followed by later improvement are both par for the course when treating Lyme disease with antibiotics.

Furthermore, since autism is generally much more severe than adult-acquired Lyme disease, it stands to reason that the cycle of worsening and improving that occurs when Lyme disease is treated with antibiotics might be much more extreme, unpredictable, and dramatic when it occurs in autistic children as opposed to when it occurs in adults suffering from Lyme disease. This may explain why researchers, despite years of trying to unravel the puzzle of how antibiotic treatment affects autistic children, have as yet been mostly stumped by the question. The observable results of antibiotic treatment in autistic children are just too erratic and unpredictable to draw meaningful, measured conclusions from.

By now you have probably noticed a statement that has been repeated throughout this book: "This data, by itself, is not conclusive, but adds supporting evidence to the Lyme-autism hypothesis." Such is also the case with the concepts we have just looked at relating to antibiotic use in autistic children. The Lyme-autism connection is not comprised of one or two incontrovertible, breakthrough facts, but instead, dozens of smaller, more subtle clues, which, when taken in aggregate, capture the gestalt of the Lyme-autism connection. The connection hypothesis is a classic example of the well-known saying that "the whole is greater than the sum of the parts."

The Primary Lyme-Autism Study

We have seen that there are numerous physicians, scientists, and researchers studying the many components of the Lyme-autism connection *separately*. There are researchers studying autism, researchers studying Lyme disease, and researchers studying various infections. Are there any researchers looking into how these separate components could be interrelated? Is anyone putting together the pieces of the puzzle to see if the completed picture looks like it supports the Lyme-autism connection?

The answer is yes. However, since this field of study is so new, not many have undertaken such a project yet. We will now take a look at the primary study that fits this description.

The most important Lyme-autism study in existence at the time of this book's publication, and the study upon which this book is largely based, was released in September, 2007, in the Medical Hypotheses Journal published by Elsevier. The study is entitled *The Association Between Tick-Borne Infections, Lyme Borreliosis and Autism Spectrum Disorders*. As noted throughout this book, a large portion of the evidence substantiating the Lyme-autism connection has been deduced and extrapolated from articles specifically on Lyme disease and articles specifically on autism, with very few articles in existence looking at both afflictions and the ways in which they may be similar or correlated. That is why the *Medical Hypotheses* article we are about to look at is so important—this study set out with the specific goal of analyzing a possible Lyme-autism connection.

Additionally, this study is important because it was authored by medical professionals and published in a peer-reviewed journal. Accordingly, it offers the credibility that is necessary in order for the Lyme-autism connection to be further studied and, eventually, possibly widely recognized.

Authors

The article was authored by the following physicians:

1. Robert C. Bransfield, MD, Department of Psychiatry, Riverview Medical Center, Red Bank, NJ, United States

2. Jeffrey S. Wulfman, MD, Department of Family Medicine, University of Vermont, Brandon, VT, United States

3. William T. Harvey, MD, Rocky Mountain Chronic Disease Specialists, Colorado Springs, CO, United States

4. Anju I. Usman, MD, True Health Medical Center, Naperville, IL, United States

The combined experience of these researchers results in a highly valuable, inter-disciplinary perspective on the Lyme-autism connection. Here is some brief background on several of the authors of the study.

Dr. Bransfield has extensive experience studying Lyme disease and has produced numerous articles on the topic. His research has contributed to a much greater understanding of the infection, specifically in the area of neurological Borreliosis. His most impactful articles include such titles as the following:

- What Causes Illness and Mental Illness?
- Microbes and Mental Illness
- Spirochetes on the Brain
- Lyme Disease and Cognitive Impairments
- Lyme, Depression, and Suicide
- Posttraumatic Stress Disorder and Infectious Encephalopathies
- Aggression and Lyme Disease
- A Tale of Two Spirochetes
- Sex and Lyme Disease
- All In Your Head?
- The Psychotropic Management of Late-Stage Lyme Disease
- Neuropsychiatric Assessment of Lyme Disease

To learn more about Dr. Bransfield's research, visit his website at www.mentalhealthandillness.com.

Dr. Wulfman is a family practice physician affiliated with the University of Vermont School of Medicine.

Dr. Harvey was well-suited for the study, given his background in chronic disease research. He has written numerous articles of interest, including, of particular note, an article entitled *Lyme disease: ancient engine of an unrecognized borreliosis pandemic?* Dr. Harvey also stays on the cutting edge of modern disease pandemics and is, at the time of this book's publication, both a board member and the chairman of the *Morgellons Research Foundation*, www.morgellons.org.

Dr. Usman brought autism expertise to the table for this study. A family physician in the Chicago area, she follows the principals of the Defeat Autism Now organization (also known as "DAN", www.defeatautismnow.com). According to her biography, Dr. Usman "has special expertise in the nuances of biochemical aberrations in children with autism spectrum disorders and teaches advanced strategies for tough cases."

Now that we have established the qualifications of the participating researchers, let's move on to examine exactly what the study set out to do, and what the findings were. We will begin with a summary of the study and then take a more thorough look at the details of the research that was performed.

Summary

(Abbreviations used in this study: TBI=Tick Borne Infection, ASD=Autism Spectrum Disorder)

1. **HYPOTHESIS**: The hypothesis upon which the researchers based the study is as follows:

   "Chronic infectious diseases, including tick-borne infections such as Borrelia burgdorferi may have direct effects, promote other infections and create a weakened, sensitized and immunologically vulnerable state during fetal development and infancy leading to increased vulnerability for developing autism spectrum disorders. A dysfunctional synergism with other predisposing and contributing factors may contribute to autism spectrum disorders..."

2. **OBSERVATION**. The study goes on to describe the people who have observed the above phenomena:

   "An association between Lyme disease (LYD) and other tick-borne infections (TBI) during fetal development and in infancy with autism, autism spectrum disorders (ASD) and autistic symptoms has been noted by numerous clinicians and parents."

3. **EVIDENCE**. The following are specific, measurable, scientifically quantifiable observations which the study relies on to support the Lyme-autism connection hypothesis:

- *Multiple cases of mothers with Lyme disease and children with autism spectrum disorders*

- *Fetal neurological abnormalities associated with tick-borne diseases*

- *Similarities between tick-borne diseases and autism spectrum disorder regarding symptoms, pathophysiology, immune reactivity, temporal lobe pathology, and brain imaging data*

- *Similar geographic distribution, and improvement in autistic symptoms from antibiotic treatment*

- *Positive serum reactivity in several studies with autistic spectrum disorder patients for Borrelia burgdorferi (22%, 26% and 20–30%) and 58% for mycoplasma*

4. **RESEARCH ORGANIZATION**. Who is gathering the data?

"A Lyme Induced Autism Foundation (LIAF) conference explored the association between Borrelia burgdorferi sensu lato (the bacterium that can cause Lyme disease and Borreliosis) as well as other tick-borne or infectious diseases and Autism Spectrum Disorders (ASD). This article was written to collate information from conference presentations on this issue with other sources that further address this association."

Details of the Study

As noted, a large portion of the study was based on observations made by parents and physicians. Both parents and physicians have observed that a great deal of symptom overlap exists between Lyme disease and autism, including such symptoms as hyperacusis, emotional detachment, mood instability, decline in speech and language, sensitivity to environmental pollutants and allergens, food intolerances, intense cravings for sugar/carbohydrates leading to symptom flareups, and adverse reactions to medications.

One of the primary supporting observations presented in the study is the shocking tendency for mothers afflicted with tick-borne diseases to give birth to ASD (autism spectrum disorders) children. Specifically, "a number of clinicians in addition to the authors have noted multiple cases of mothers with tick-borne infections and children with ASD, infants infected with tick-borne infections who had ASD or autistic symptoms, children infected with tick-borne infections with autistic symptoms and children with ASD who acquired tick-borne infections and displayed an exacerbation of ASD symptoms."

Additionally, the authors note that patients suffering from ASD and tick-borne infections have inflammatory bowel disorders and gastrointestinal symptoms. In both diseases, gastrointestinal symptoms have shown improvement with the use of antibiotics.

Earlier in the book, you read about the scientific evidence that the Lyme disease infection can be transferred from mother to child during pregnancy. According to the *Medical Hypotheses* article, the observations of one of the nation's current leading pediatric Lyme specialists, Dr. Charles Ray Jones, confirms this phenomenon: "Jones et al. estimates he has seen approximately 300 cases of gestational TBI. All of the mothers had untreated or inadequately treated TBI either prior to or during pregnancy." Of the more than 102 childhood cases Dr. Jones analyzed, 9% had been diagnosed with autism and 56% had been diagnosed with attention deficit disorder.

Dr. Jones found that many of his patients suffered from irritability, anger and rage, anxiety, depression, obsessive-compulsive disorder, suicidal thoughts, headache, vertigo, developmental delays, seizure disorders, poor memory, dyslexia, and gastrointestinal symptoms. Again, all of these symptoms are shared in common between Lyme disease and ASD.

During his research, Dr. Jones discovered that 66 mothers with Lyme disease who were appropriately treated with antibiotics prior to conception and during their entire pregnancies gave birth to healthy infants.

What about objective testing? In modern times, with modern medical technology, why can we not find tick-borne infections in autistic children via laboratory testing? Well, we can and we do. Pilot studies that test ASD children for tick-borne infections have been conducted. Aristo Vojdani, Ph.D., reported at the 2007 LIA Foundation conference that he tested autistic children from various clinics in California, New York, New Jersey, and Connecticut. 22% (12 of 54) samples tested IgG and IgM positive for Borrelia via Immunosciences Lab (www.immuno-sci-lab.com).

An additional study supervised by LIA Foundation tested the blood of 19 children with ASD and immune dysfunction, along with five normal controls. Laboratory testing was conducted by IGeneX (www.igenex.com). 26% of ASD children were positive in comparison to zero percent of controls.

The results of other tests of ASD children were also presented at the 2007 LIA Foundation conference. Warren Levin, MD, tested nine ASD patients in 2003 and all were positive for Borrelia. Garth Nicolson, Ph.D., of the Institute for Molecular Medicine (www.immed.org) tested 48 ASD patients with forensic PCR and Southern Blot confirmation. More than 20% tested positive for Borrelia, and a high percentage also tested positive for co-infections.

The presence of infections in patients with tick-borne infections and ASD is not where the laboratory test similarities end. In fact, in addition to finding Borrelia and co-infections in both disease groups, numerous other biochemical similarities also exist. Examples include overlap in the following areas: "Disorders of oxidoreductive system in CSF and serum, increases of superoxide dismutase, increased glutathione peroxidase activity, increased concentration of serum malondialdehyde, decreased glutathione, alterations in the activities of antioxidant enzymes such as superoxide dismutase and glutathione peroxidase, altered glutathione levels and homocysteine/methionine metabolism, increased malondialdehyde levels and reduced glutathione."

Remarkably, similarities in laboratory results go even further. In addition to biochemical similarities and overlap in the presence of specific infections, Lyme patients also share in common similar brain imaging results with ASD patients. Similarities include significant temporal lobe dysfunction, white matter encephalopathy, and increased activity of both the thalamus and cortex.

To this point we have looked at what the study says about similarities in symptom presentation, gestational transfer, and laboratory testing. Let's move on and see what the authors of the *Medical Hypotheses* study have to say about similarities in epidemiological findings. Epidemiology is the study of disease distribution in a population. If Lyme disease and ASD are unrelated, it would be expected that their incidence and epidemiology would also show no correlation. In the authors' words, "A causal association is suggested if the geographical patterns of ASD and BI/TBI overlap and are co-morbid more than would be expected by random association."

So, is there a causal association? According to the study, "In a geostatistical review of CDC and IDEA statistics, 10 out of the top

15 states overlap for the incidence of autism and Lyme disease (MN, ME, MA, MD, CT, WI, RI, NJ, PA, VA)." Research relied on in the writing of this book agrees (see Chapter 6 for additional, in-depth statistical analysis of Lyme-autism epidemiology).

It is critical to note also that the authors of the study found numerous other infections accompanying the Lyme infection (known as "co-infections"). The most important of these are bartonella, mycoplasma, babesia, ehrlichia, and leptospirosis. In some cases, these coinfections may actually be just as, or more significant than, Borrelia itself. In most cases, it is the combination of Borrelia with these co-infections—the "infection stew," as we have called it—that leads to the most severe damage.

Finally, to conclude our look at this study, it is important to note that the multiplicity of autism cannot be forgotten. The autistic condition is caused by multiple factors, not a single dysfunction or single infection. This important point is summed up in the *Medical Hypotheses* study:

> *"Most commonly human diseases are caused by the interaction of environmental insults and susceptibility genes. Many of the susceptibility genes result in human response to environmental factors and infection. Environmental insults contributing to ASD may include a complex interaction with infections, heavy metals, biotoxins, allergens, nutritional excesses/deficits and possibly vaccines."*

In a book on the Lyme-autism connection, it is critical that readers recognize the multifactorial nature of autism and, when formulating a treatment plan, recognize that numerous strategies must be incorporated. The Lyme-autism connection does not state that Lyme disease is the only underlying cause of autism, but instead, that Lyme disease might be one of *many* underlying causes.

Open Studies

The following two studies are currently underway in examining the link between autism and infections:

1. Brian Fallon, MD, working for the Columbia University Lyme Disease Research Center, is currently conducting a study entitled *Developmental Delay and Lyme Disease in Children: An Epidemiologic Study*. According to the Columbia University website (www.columbia-lyme.org), the study has the following characteristics:

   Participants: Children with Lyme disease & Autism from New Jersey and Connecticut

   Goals: To understand more about the association between LD and developmental delay and developmental regression

   Status of study: Underway. As this is a population-based study, we are not recruiting individual patients.

   Principal Investigator: Brian A. Fallon, MD

   To learn more about the study, visit www.columbia-lyme.org.

2. The NIH (National Institutes of Health) is currently examining the potential benefit of using minocycline to treat autism. According to the NIH, *"researchers will examine the use of the antibiotic minocycline to measure its usefulness in treating regressive autism. Past research suggests that autism may be linked with changes in the immune response that cause inflammation in the brain. Minocycline has known anti-inflammatory effects and has been shown to be helpful in other brain disorders such as Huntington's disease."*

   The NIH study is interesting for a number of reasons, and it is worth pausing here for a minute to conduct a deeper analysis. The NIH claims it is performing this study because previous studies have shown that minocycline has a surprising and dramatic ability to control idiopathic neurological conditions. The NIH is attributing the possible benefit of minocycline to its anti-inflammatory effects, yet there is a growing compilation of evidence which suggests that this may not be the case, and that the benefit gleaned from minocycline in idiopathic diseases such as Huntington's Disease is not due to anti-inflammatory effects, but instead, the targeting of stealth pathogens infecting the central nervous system. Consider the following facts.

a. Numerous anti-inflammatory drugs are available, including various kinds of steroidal and non-steroidal choices, yet historically, minocycline (an antibiotic), has outperformed them all in controlling or curing idiopathic neurological conditions. Are the antibiotic properties of minocycline merely coincidental to its anti-inflammatory properties, or are the antibiotic properties actually responsible for the healing activity? Assuming the beneficial actions of minocycline are anti-inflammatory instead of antibiotic in nature is, again, guilty of the logical fallacy "begging the question." In other words, instead of rationally considering the evidence, the researchers are prematurely integrating their assumed conclusions into their premises.

b. Minocycline is one of the most effective oral antibiotics for treating infections in the central nervous system. In comparison with other oral antibiotics, minocycline has excellent blood-brain-barrier penetration, and is highly fat soluble (the brain is comprised of fatty tissues). Additionally, in comparison with its cousins doxycycline and tetracycline, minocycline shows five times the killing activity and five times the tissue penetration. Again, are these astounding antibiotic qualities merely a coincidence—an irrelevant property of the drug—or are they the properties which are exerting the beneficial effect? While the NIH contends that these astounding antibiotic actions of minocycline are nothing but a coincidence, logic seems to disagree.

c. The fact that the NIH knows that inflammation is occurring in the autistic brain, yet does not recognize the possibility that an infection is the root cause, is simply illogical. In most cases of non-traumatic brain inflammation, infection is high on the list of differential diagnoses and suspected culprits. If someone presented at the emergency room with brain inflammation, the first tests run would be those looking for viral or bacterial meningitis and/or encephalopathy. The mainstream medical establishment even recognizes— and respects—chronic forms of these brain infections. So why is it so difficult to accept the possibility that brain inflammation in autism might be due to a similar bacterial or viral pathogenesis?

The above studies are not conclusive yet because they are not complete. While we wait for the results to be published, let's move on to examine another overlap between Lyme disease and autism which further supports the Lyme-autism hypothesis: symptom overlap.

Chapter 5
Connecting the Dots: Common Symptomology

Symptom similarities between Lyme disease and autism, especially in children, are astounding. Obviously, symptom similarity alone is not a strong enough scientific indicator to implicate Lyme disease in the autism epidemic. However, when considered within the framework of the other arguments presented in this book, symptom similarity becomes an important, central piece of the puzzle.

This chapter was written with three primary goals. First, we will look at the diagnostic procedures used in classifying mental illnesses. Then we will show that a Lyme disease diagnosis overlaps with numerous other mental disorders. Finally, we will show that an autism diagnosis not only overlaps with a variety of different mental illnesses as well, but that they happen to be, in many cases, the same mental illnesses which overlap with Lyme disease. Additionally, the chapter will also cover various data which support the above three points.

Symptoms vs. Syndromes

At first glance, the obvious question to ask in this chapter is whether or not the symptoms of Lyme disease overlap with the symptoms of autism. As you will see, however, this question is much too broad. You will see that Lyme disease is known as the "great imitator" because it can mimic dozens of seemingly unrelated health problems. Lyme disease symptoms overlap with just about every mental illness, so it is not very impressive to show that they also overlap with autism.

For this reason, we will instead take a narrower look at the symptom similarities between Lyme disease and autism, and delve further into analyzing the overlap. Namely, we will not look at individual symptoms the diseases share in common, but instead at entire disease syndromes which the two diseases share in common. For example, we will go further than to just say "Lyme disease and autism both cause headaches." Rather, we will say that "Lyme disease and autism both manifest as schizophrenia." A headache is an individual symptom, while schizophrenia is a complex syndrome.

For our purpose of further analyzing the Lyme-autism connection, it is more helpful to look at overlapping disease syndromes instead of just overlapping symptoms because disease syndromes are much more complex, specific, and isolated than are individual symptoms. Many things can cause a headache, such as fatigue, a bad lunch, or a fight with a spouse. So, demonstrating that Lyme disease and autism both cause headaches does not add much support to the Lyme-autism connection. Schizophrenia, on the other hand, is not caused by many factors, and cannot be confused with simple triggers like a bad hamburger or emotional stress. By narrowing the comparison down to specific disease syndromes, we can build a much stronger case for the Lyme-autism connection.

Blurred Lines Between Disease Labels

In order to show that both Lyme disease and autism share in common numerous disease syndromes, we must first accept the fact that the diagnostic lines are blurred between autism, Lyme disease, and numerous other mental illnesses, leading to somewhat arbitrary and meaningless guidelines for diagnosing the diseases. For example, someone diagnosed with the label "schizophrenia" may in fact be suffering from Lyme disease, autism, or both. "Schizophrenia" is not a disease; instead it is a disease *presentation*. The label *schizophrenia* says nothing about the *reason* for the disease, or the cause, but instead simply says that a given person is suffering from a collection of physiologic and symptomatic dysfunctions.

It is important to keep this in mind as you think about Lyme disease, autism, and the list of mimicking diseases. You have to ask yourself, "Does the disease label in question tell me anything about what is actually causing this health problem?" Understanding that many of the disease labels used by conventional medicine are actually not indicative of the cause of the disease will help you learn how to adjust your thinking process and see that many "diseases" do not in fact have established, defined boundaries separating them from other "diseases," but are instead simply a melting pot of symptomatic and physiological characteristics.

Why is this important? Let's again use the example of a headache. When someone says, "I have a headache," you would never jump to a conclusion about what is causing the headache unless you knew more about the person's current circumstances. A headache is not a disease in and of itself; instead it is a list of symptomatic and physiologic properties, namely, pain in the head, and typically, inflammation in the head. We all know that many things can cause headaches, hence, if someone mentions their headache, the next thing you might try to do is play detective to discover what is causing the headache. You might ask the person what they ate for lunch, how much sleep they are getting, or what is happening at work. You would never assume that the cause of their headache is the headache itself. Headaches always have underlying, root causes.

In the same way, if someone has schizophrenia or autism, you should train your mind to play the same detective role. Schizophrenia and autism are no more the cause of a health problem than is a headache. Instead, schizophrenia and autism are just labels for a set of symptomatic and physiologic characteristics. When you begin to adopt this way of thinking, you can see that the lines between various diseases can easily become blurred.

When autism is seen as a set of symptoms rather than a defined "disease," it leaves a lot more room for questions—questions which can ultimately lead to a better understanding of the disease and its cause(s). Do not passively accept a diagnosis of autism as the final description of your child's health. You should empower yourself to play detective and get to the bottom of the symptoms, instead of simply accepting the diagnosis and giving up.

If you think about Lyme disease and autism as separate diseases, with distinct boundaries, then the Lyme-autism connection seems improbable. However, if you think of the two diseases accurately, as nothing more than arbitrary labels which encompass a grouping of symptoms, some of which overlap, then the question arises and must be answered: what is the *root cause* of the disease syndromes? Is the root cause potentially the same?

Now, a clarifying point is in order here. Some diseases certainly do include causative factors in their label. For example, strep throat is caused by...strep bacteria in the throat. The disease label "strep throat" is one which is accurate in its description of causality. Similarly, Lyme disease is caused by Lyme disease bacteria (the scientific name for which is Borrelia burgdorferi). So, when we are looking at the Lyme-autism connection, what we are really asking is whether or not autism shares the same root cause as Lyme disease, namely, a Borrelia infection.

Ok, so this all sounds good in theory, but where is the evidence? Let's now turn our attention to several scientific studies which provide objective substantiation for the theory we just talked about—the theory that mental disorders have blurred diagnostic lines.

Lyme Disease: The Great Imitator

To substantiate the theory that disease labels are relatively arbitrary and have blurred defining lines, let's begin by looking at Lyme disease and the many diseases which it mimics.

The Journal of Neuropsychiatry in 2001 published an article in which it was stated that "Children with Lyme disease have...cognitive and psychiatric disturbances...resulting in psycho-social and academic impairments." According to Dr. Frederic Blanc, of the University of Strasbourg, France, "The neurological and psychiatric manifestations of Borrelia are so numerous that it is called the 'new great imitator.' Every part of the nervous system can be involved: from central to peripheral."

It is difficult to convey just how broad and diverse Lyme disease symptoms can be. As the "new great imitator" (Syphilis was considered the original great imitator), Lyme disease mimics dozens of seemingly unrelated illnesses, from physical disorders such as chronic fatigue syndrome and arthritis, to psychiatric disorders including schizophrenia, obsessive compulsive disorder, Tourette syndrome, depression, bipolar disorder, and more. According to psychiatrists at Columbia University, as published in 1994 in the American Journal of Psychiatry:

"Lyme disease can trigger a broad range of psychiatric reactions, including paranoia, dementia, schizophrenia, bipolar disorder, panic attacks, major depression, anorexia nervosa and obsessive–compulsive disorder."

As you can see, Lyme disease is often the root cause of a long list of diseases. In these cases, there is in fact zero separation between the seemingly distinct diseases on the list—the lines are blurred beyond recognition. A variety of mental disorders can potentially all have the same root cause.

Antiquated belief that Lyme disease is characterized by a limited set of mostly benign symptoms is rapidly being replaced by modern, increasingly accurate models of Lyme disease symptomology that encompass a vast diversity of symptomology in numerous body systems. So, if you are doubtful that a simple bacterial infection can cause such diverse symptoms as are present in autism, be forewarned—Lyme disease is a highly advanced neuropsychiatric disease with complicated and poorly understood effects on the brain. The combination of wide-ranging symptoms and the prevalence of false-negative laboratory test results means that Lyme disease may be one of the most rampant, yet under-diagnosed, infections on the planet. And, when the Lyme infection occurs in the womb, a new set of variables and complexities are introduced to the scene which further broaden the potential neurological effects of Lyme disease.

Still, the fact that Lyme disease is a great imitator is nothing worth writing home about—this has become accepted science in both mainstream and alternative medicine. Therefore, we will not belabor this point here. To learn more about Lyme disease as a great imitator, read Appendix B and consult available Lyme disease literature.

The real point we are tracking down in this chapter is not merely the fact that Lyme disease shares blurred lines with many mental illnesses, but, more importantly, the fact that autism also shares blurred lines with a variety of mental disorders. Even more important yet is the paramount question of whether or not Lyme disease and autism share blurred lines with *the same set* of mental illnesses.

Autism: The Next Great Imitator?

You may be surprised to learn that just as Lyme disease is a great imitator, so also is autism.

Many autistic people have a broad range of psychological symptoms, not just those few which have historically defined "classic" autism. Autism is currently being re-defined as a multi-systemic, multi-factorial disease. In this section, we will examine some of the science surrounding autism as a great imitator. For each of the scientific studies below, we will note their relevance to the Lyme-autism connection.

Swedish researchers have observed a fascinating overlap between symptoms of autism and other mental illnesses. In 2004, the Department of Child and Adolescent Psychiatry, at Göteborg University, Sweden, published findings in the *Journal of Neural Transmission* indicating that patients suffering from autism also sometimes have symptoms of schizophrenia, bipolar disorder, and attention-deficit/hyperactivity disorder (AD/HD). The Swedish researchers don't offer an explanation for this symptom overlap, but they do acknowledge it, and conclude their study by stating that "Current diagnostic criteria have to be revised to acknowledge the co-morbidity of autism with bipolar disorder, AD/HD, schizophrenia, and other psychotic diseases."

The connection: Of the mental illnesses which Lyme disease mimics, schizophrenia, bipolar disorder, and attention-deficit/hyperactivity disorder are at the top of the list.

Researchers at the University of Michigan published a study in 2004 in the *Journal of Autism and Developmental Disorders* which concluded with the following statement: "This study lends support to the validity of depression as a distinct condition in some children with autism/PDD and suggests that, as in the normal population, autistic children who suffer from depression are more likely to have a family history of depression."

The connection: These findings are significant for two reasons: first, the study indicates that depression is part of the autism complex of symptoms, and second, this depression can be found in family history. Both of these points are true of Lyme disease, as well.

In London, similar conclusions are being reached. The Genetic and Developmental Psychiatry Research Centre published in 1998 a study entitled "Autism, affective and other psychiatric disorders: patterns of familial aggregation." The report was released by Cambridge University Press in the Journal of Psychological Medicine. In addition to finding a correlation between familial mental disorders and autism, researchers also discovered that "Individuals with a singular diagnosis of obsessive-compulsive disorder were more likely to exhibit autistic-like social and communication impairments."

The connection: This finding is fascinating because it tells us that not only does autism involve symptoms of other, previously believed separate diseases, but the converse of this is also true; that those separate diseases also sometimes include symptoms known to occur in autism. This further blurs the lines between different mental disorders. This is another piece of the puzzle that shatters the previous belief that autism is completely distinct and separate from other psychiatric diseases. Modern medicine likes to put these diseases in their own neatly organized, unrelated files, but reality just won't comply with such an organizational strategy.

City of Hope National Medical Center in California published findings that link autism and Tourette syndrome. Researchers found that "there is an intimate genetic, neuropathologic relatedness between some cases of [autism] and Tourette syndrome." Additionally, these researchers noted frequent family groupings of the two afflictions, with obsessive compulsive disorder also showing up frequently.

The connection: The Lancet in 1998 published a study linking Lyme disease with Tourette syndrome. A 4-year old boy developed typical Tourette symptoms and was subsequently diagnosed with Lyme disease by ELISA IgG antibody testing. Upon antibiotic treatment, all symptoms resolved. From the Lancet: "Rapid efficacy of antibiotic treatment followed by a decrease in Borrelia-specific antibody titres suggests that the multiple motor and vocal tics [in this 4-year old boy] were at least partially caused by the tertiary stage of Borreliosis." Therefore, both autism and Lyme disease share in common blurred lines with Tourette syndrome.

The lines between autism and other mental disorders are further blurred when considering the methods used to diagnose autism. This is an important area to examine because the diagnostic model used in categorizing childhood mental disorders is the primary determinant of the next twenty or more years of treatment decisions. Consider this carefully—if a child is diagnosed with autism but Lyme disease is really the root problem, then parents will spend thousands (or maybe millions) of dollars, thousands of hours, and incalculable stress, pursuing the wrong course(s) of treatment. Hence, proper diagnostic procedures, or at least, proper understanding of the limitations of modern diagnostic capabilities, is essential for ensuring that a lifetime of energy is focused in the right direction. This statement is substantiated by the experiences of numerous mothers, whose stories appear in Appendix E. These mothers only received desirable treatment results after discovering the Lyme infection in their children. Prior to the discovery, they wasted incalculable time, energy and money chasing palliative treatments.

Alarmingly, the diagnostic model used for autism can be relatively unreliable. The Indiana University School of Medicine in 1971 evaluated 5 diagnostic systems designed to differentiate infantile autism and early childhood schizophrenia and published their findings in the *Journal of Autism and Developmental Disorders*. Diagnostic scores from 44 children were examined. Some of the five diagnostic systems contradicted the others, leading to a confusing and disturbing debate about the definitions of autism and schizophrenia. So similar are the two diseases that the lines between them become blurred when using these diagnostic systems, and the results of the diagnostic procedures become relatively meaningless. Obviously, diagnostic systems have improved exponentially since 1971. However, even today, the same symptom similarities exist between autism and schizophrenia, resulting in debate and disagreement about proper courses of treatment for the two disorders, not to mention heated arguments between parents and physicians about which treatments are most logical to pursue. Modern medicine's appearance of having everything figured out, with white-coated, authoritative doctors passing down final diagnostic decrees to parents, is riddled with an uncertain and ambiguous past.

The tendency to over-compartmentalize diseases without sufficient data is not limited to just the commercial medical industry—non-profit research organizations dedicated to healing schizophrenia and autism also suffer the effects of arbitrarily separating autism from schizophrenia when conducting research and presenting information. The reality is that autism and schizophrenia are intimately related, and only when this fact is accounted for will true breakthrough occur in the research of the two conditions. Autism and schizophrenia are not two separate entities like the colors black and white. They resemble more closely a shade of grey, mixing some amount of black and some amount of white. When researchers only look at the black, they miss the big picture, and when they only look at white, they don't see all of the facts. Only when shades of grey are acknowledged, will the mechanisms behind the afflictions become more apparent.

Any parent with an autistic child knows that their child exhibits a wide array of symptoms and that no two days are alike. Unlike high cholesterol or diabetes, which are fairly constant disorders with very few variations in symptoms and presentation, autism is a wildly variable condition that seems to follow no particular pattern or predictable course.

Thus far in this chapter, we have worked to establish that not only do Lyme disease and autism act like great imitators, but the diseases which they imitate happen to be the *same diseases*— namely, mental disorders such as schizophrenia, obsessive compulsive disorder, depression, Tourette syndrome, AD/HD, and others. Although this overlap in associated disease syndromes (and, more broadly, associated individual symptoms) is not sufficient evidence to stand alone as the foundation for the Lyme-autism connection, this observation is, again, one more piece of the puzzle.

It really is shocking and insightful to discover that Lyme disease and autism are separated by much less space than medical schools and textbooks teach. If these broad similarities are not explained by an underlying Lyme disease infection, then what is the explanation? Isn't it a bit improbable that two supposedly separate diseases are so intimately related in so many ways?

The ven diagram on the following page illustrates these concepts.

The center circle of this ven diagram shows that both Lyme disease and autism share many symptoms in common with other mental illnesses.

The important fact here is that Lyme disease and autism share symptoms in common not just with many illnesses, but with the <u>same set</u> of many illnesses.

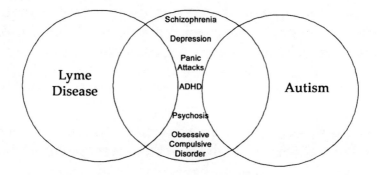

Lyme Disease

Schizophrenia

Depression

Panic Attacks

ADHD

Autism

Psychosis

Obsessive Compulsive Disorder

VEN DIAGRAM: SYMPTOM OVERLAP

Before concluding this chapter, we will briefly introduce one more area of overlap: autoimmunity.

Autoimmunity

Lyme disease and autism not only share numerous similarities with regard to psychiatric symptoms and syndromes, but also autoimmunity.

The number of studies linking both Lyme disease and autism to autoimmune dysfunction is vast, encompassing dozens of published articles released by several research institutions. For specific studies, visit MEDLINE at www.ncbi.nlm.nih.gov/PubMed and search for keywords *autism autoimmune* and *lyme disease autoimmune*. At the time of this writing, the first search string yielded 86 studies and the second string yielded 123 studies.

The fact that Lyme disease and autism share autoimmunity in common is, of course, fascinating, and lends credit to the Lyme-autism hypothesis. However, the link becomes even stronger in light of the fact that new research is revealing that many autoimmune disorders are caused by stealth infections. Recent research has found that treatments aimed at eradicating stealth infections happen to also provide relief, and in some cases, remission or cure, for autoimmune diseases.

One such cutting-edge treatment is the Marshall Protocol, discussed at length in *The Top 10 Lyme Disease Treatments*. The Marshall Protocol is significant in this context because it defines and reveals the mechanism by which symptoms of autoimmunity can really be an indication of underlying infection. Patients experiencing healing on the Marshall Protocol suffer from a wide range of autoimmune disorders—and healing is taking place via the anti-infective treatments that comprise the protocol. Autoimmunity is defined as the body attacking its own cells. But why would it do that? The new, prevailing theory is that there is a stealth infection inhabiting body tissues and when the immune system attempts to attack that infection, it mistakenly attacks its own proteins which might look similar to the proteins that compose the infectious microorganisms. This new theory of autoimmunity is gaining momentum.

It shouldn't surprise us that autoimmunity is involved in Lyme disease. After all, Lyme disease is known to be caused by an infection. However, what about autism? Why is there autoimmunity in autism? Is there an underlying infection? If, in fact, autoimmunity is caused by an infectious process, then the autoimmune link between Lyme disease and autism becomes quite telling and is, yet again, just another piece of the puzzle.

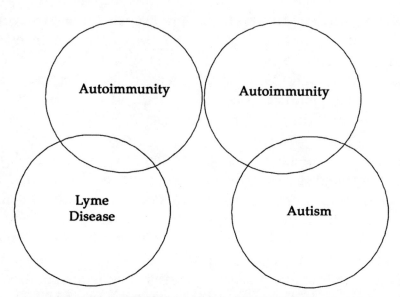

The above ven diagram represents the similar, but not significantly related, conditions of autism and Lyme disease given that autoimmunity does not have infectious etiology.

The below ven diagram shows that if the autoimmunity involved in Lyme disease and autism is in fact caused by infection, then the two conditions may be more closely related.

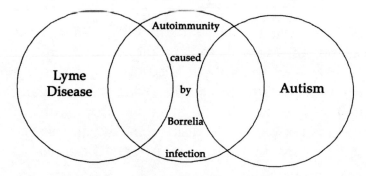

VEN DIAGRAM: AUTOIMMUNITY AND INFECTIONS

The ven diagram on the opposing page illustrates that an infectious root cause of autoimmunity in Lyme disease and autism results in the diseases being more closely related to one another.

(Note: The Marshall Protocol is experimental and has not been proven safe for children. This protocol may not be an appropriate treatment for autistic children. Consult a physician before using the Marshall Protocol or any other treatment discussed in this book.)

Where the Rubber Meets the Road

Hopefully, this chapter has given you a new perspective on childhood developmental disorders. Remember, if your child gets diagnosed with any of the disease labels we have just looked at, do not be satisfied with the diagnosis. Being diagnosed with attention deficit disorder is like being diagnosed with a headache. A headache is not a diagnosis, it is a symptom. A headache is the beginning of the diagnostic journey, not the end. The same can be said of attention deficit disorder.

The minute you start treating your child's attention deficit disorder (or autism, or schizophrenia, or fill-in-the-blank disorder) as if it is a complete diagnosis, you are beginning a losing battle. Why? The reason is logical and simple. Since these disease labels do not factor in the true cause(s) of the disease (whatever the cause(s) may be), the only treatment modern medicine can offer you is palliative treatment. Palliative treatment is that which covers symptoms instead of addressing cause. The word palliative is derived from the Latin word palliare, which means "to cloak."

Antidepressant drugs are an example of a palliative treatment, and, not surprisingly, antidepressant drugs are the treatment most often given for childhood developmental disorders. Other palliative drugs include anti-psychotic, anti-anxiety, and sedative. These drugs only temporarily snuff out the symptoms of the underlying problem. And, these drugs have ghastly, brutal side effects of which the public is becoming increasingly aware—such as aggressive behavior, suicidal thoughts and ideation, and decline in intellect. Are these horrendous side effects justified given that the drugs are not even addressing the cause of the disease?

Most of the autism treatment programs and centers in the United States (at least among mainstream medicine) do nothing but offer palliative, or "behavioral" treatment. The government, non-profit research organizations, and parents spend millions of dollars on palliative treatments for childhood developmental disorders. What would happen if some of that money were actually spent on what really matters; that is, trying to locate and treat the cause? Would you offer physical therapy to someone suffering from a broken leg, or would you repair the broken leg?

Now that you are equipped with knowledge, and you know that childhood developmental disorders do in fact have underlying, scientific, physiological causes (even though these causes are sometimes elusive and difficult to isolate), you can begin to play detective with your child and treat the causes, not the symptoms, of their disease. Palliative treatments are useful to increase quality of life during the discovery process. But the palliative treatments themselves are *not* the end goal.

Maybe your child's disorder is caused by an imbalance of intestinal microflora. In this case, you might consider using probiotics, diet, and herbs to correct the problem. Or maybe, it is mercury poisoning, for which you could use chelation. Or possibly, your child's disorder is caused by food allergies, which you might alleviate by an elimination diet. Or, as this book proposes, maybe your child's autism is caused by Lyme disease, in which case you may decide to undergo Lyme treatment. Whatever the underlying cause, the thought pattern is the same: you, as the parent, must step up to the plate, take responsibility, reject the "diagnosis" your child was given, and search for the underlying cause.

A good friend of mine (Bryan) suffered from migraine headaches for years. She drained her bank account trying the strongest painkillers and anti-migraine medications available. She endured the side effects of powerful, dangerous pharmaceuticals. She only received minimal relief, and suffered greatly. One day, a thinking physician inquired about her diet and discovered that she consumed diet soda pop once or twice a day, every day of her life. In fact, if she ran out of soda, she would make a special trip to the store to replenish her stock. After she objected vehemently, he finally convinced her to go without the soda for a few weeks. Bingo! The headaches disappeared, almost overnight. The palliative, symptom-covering painkillers were not the answer (although they did make a few CEOs and stockholders richer). Eliminating the root cause was the answer.

I do not want to oversimplify childhood developmental disorders. In most cases, the detective work necessary is much more difficult than the experience my friend had with her headaches. However, you owe it to yourself and your child to at least try the detective strategy. In the best case scenario, you will cure your child, and in the worst case scenario, you will at least become educated about your son or daughter's body, and provide him or her with some level of relief, however minor. But most importantly, taking a detective approach will ensure that you are doing absolutely everything you can to be a good parent.

You, as a thinking, caring, intelligent parent, have what it takes to be a detective and to reject the superficial diagnosis given by a doctor whose thinking is victim of the dogmatic, palliative treatment paradigm that currently rules American medicine.

Chapter 6
Connecting the Dots: Geographic Distribution and Incidence

Finally, after reviewing all of the other evidence supporting the Lyme-autism connection, it is time to look at the similarities between geographic distribution and chronological occurrence of Lyme disease and autism. This is the final piece of the puzzle which this book will address.

The Lyme-autism connection is a relatively new, unexplored area of research, so any statistical data we can find and analyze should be valued at a premium due to its scarcity. Both Lyme disease and autism are highly elusive, complicated, poorly understood diseases, and data on these two diseases is not only scarce, but also difficult to interpret and derive meaning from. The multi-phase, multi-systemic, masquerading properties of both conditions make their respective epidemiological study increasingly difficult and confusing.

Why is the analysis of these diseases so confounding? To answer this question, let's compare Lyme disease and autism with a comparatively simple health problem: a broken femur. There is nothing complex or confusing about a broken femur. It would be relatively easy to analyze how many times a broken femur occurs in a given population, whether its occurrence is increasing or decreasing, and whether or not common treatments effectively heal the broken bone. You could accomplish such an analysis by taking steps as simple as looking at hospital records, interviewing orthopedic physicians, and counting the number of femur surgeries that take place in a given year. If you wanted to know whether or not playing soccer increases your risk of a broken femur, this would also be quite easy to determine by means of common data-gathering practices and statistical analysis.

Lyme disease and autism present a much more complicated picture. Even if you analyze each disease individually (instead of trying to find a correlation between them), the picture is cloudy and difficult. Let's take Lyme disease, for example. After having read Appendices A and B, you will understand the ambiguity involved in properly diagnosing and tracking Lyme disease cases. Was there a tick bite? If so, was it memorable, or was the tick a nymph-stage (young) tick which is only the size of the head of a needle and invisible due to its transparent color? Did the patient in question test positive for Lyme disease or were they one of the many people who experience false-negative test results? Did the person get misdiagnosed with any number of mimicking conditions, resulting in their case of Lyme disease not being counted at all? Are the physicians in the person's city of residence trained to look for Lyme disease, or are they similar to the majority of U.S. physicians who fail to report active cases of Lyme disease due to their ignorance of the infection? Does the patient in question suffer from a mental illness which no one has identified as possible Lyme disease? Was the infection transferred to the patient before birth, in which case it may never be identified due to the conspicuous absence of the expected tick bite?

Autism is not much simpler. At what age did it develop? Which type of autism is it? What other factors are involved?

Both Lyme disease and autism are complicated enough when analyzed individually. When you attempt to look at the conditions together and how they may relate to one another, the difficulty increases exponentially.

At this point you might be wondering why we are pointing out all of the reasons why we will never be able to understand the Lyme-autism connection. If it is so complicated and ambiguous, why was this book even written? Well, actually, the reason we are painting such a muddled picture here is not to devalue the data presented in this book, but instead, to help you see the premium value of the statistical information and data which we *do* currently have. In an area of research in which knowledge is so scarce, the discovery of useful data should be considered very important. Statistical information regarding broken femurs is a dime a dozen, but statistical information relating to the Lyme-autism connection should be given due attention and be carefully examined.

That is why this chapter of the book is so important. The data in this chapter, by itself, has the power to render the Lyme-autism connection either implausible or plausible. The question we will ask is, Does the data provide a foundation—or at least, the underpinnings of a foundation—for the Lyme-autism connection, or does the data indicate that the connection is unlikely?

Let's get down to business and look at the data.

The Correlation Coefficient

In this chapter, we will be using correlation coefficient to analyze two sets of data:

1. The number of cases of Lyme disease and autism reported from 1993-2006 in the United States without respect to geography.

2. The number of cases of Lyme disease and autism reported in each state in the United States in the year 2006.

The purpose of comparing Lyme disease cases and autism cases chronologically (#1 above) and geographically (#2 above) is to determine whether or not objective statistical analysis supports a correlation between Lyme disease and autism cases. After all, if such an analysis is not supportive of the connection, then all the ink on all the pages of this book is largely irrelevant.

Before looking at the data, a quick crash course on correlation coefficient is in order. First, the definition of correlation:

> "A statistical relation between two or more variables such that systematic changes in the value of one variable are accompanied by systematic changes in the other."

Now, the definition of correlation coefficient:

> "A statistic representing how closely two variables co-vary; it can vary from -1 (perfect negative correlation) through 0 (no correlation) to +1 (perfect positive correlation)."

(Definitions according to Princeton University). Essentially, correlation coefficient is used to place a quantifiable measurement on correlation.

Correlation coefficient is interpreted to mean that for any given set of data, there is either a small, medium, or large correlation, as illustrated in Table C1 (for the sake of simplicity, we will ignore negative correlation coefficient values). It should be noted, however, that correlation coefficient must be interpreted in context—for example, a given correlation coefficient may have a completely different meaning when comparing calibration of precision instruments in comparison with the analysis of social behaviors, or other less precise areas of measurement.

In statistics, correlation coefficient is the standard tool for analyzing two sets of data to determine their relative levels of dependence or independence.

Table C1	
Significance (Strength)	Correlation Coefficient
None	0.0 to 0.1
Small	0.1 to 0.3
Medium	0.3 to 0.5
Large	0.5 to 1.0

While the mathematical formula used to determine correlation coefficient is quite complicated—and far beyond the scope of this book—understanding the significance of correlation coefficient is very simple. In short, correlation coefficient tells us whether two sets of data are related to one another.

Let's look at two brief examples to see how correlation coefficient works.

The first example is a basketball game. Every time a player scores a basket, the scoreboard shows an increase of two points (we will assume that no three-point shots are made in this game). This scenario is represented in the following table:

Baskets Scored During Game	Number of Points Added to Scoreboard
1	2
2	4
3	6
4	8

Common sense tells us that there should be a strong correlation—in fact, a perfect correlation—between the above two sets of data (the number of baskets scored and the number of points displayed on the scoreboard). After all, it is definitely predictable that making baskets will cause the scoreboard to increase. And common sense is correct! When you run the numbers in the table through the correlation coefficient mathematical function, the result is a perfect score of 1. This means that there is a perfect correlation between the two sets of variables. We can be 100% certain that the next time a basket is scored, the scoreboard will increase by two points.

Of course, just because there is a perfect correlation, does not mean there is a causative relationship. The ball falling through the hoop does not actually *cause* the scorekeeper's finger to push the button on the score-keeping machine. However, there exists a *practical* causative relationship to the extent that, under normal circumstances, we can be completely certain that scoring a basket will cause the scoreboard to jump two points.

In the second example, we will look at two variables which are not correlated. We will examine the average daily temperature in the city of Bozeman, Montana, for each month of the year in 2007, and compare that data with the average closing price per share of Yahoo! stock during the same period.

Month	Average Daily Temperature in Montana	Yahoo! Stock Share Price
January	22.19	26.21
February	28.79	28.40
March	40.90	29.34
April	44.32	31.43
May	54.56	29.34

June	62.08	27.90
July	74.63	27.28
August	67.11	24.13
September	56.88	24.21
October	47.93	23.31
November	34.00	28.81
December	12.50	26.15

The correlation coefficient of these two sets of data is .14, which, as you will recall from Table C1, is a small, and almost insignificant, correlation. This is, of course, what you would expect— there is no reason to believe that the performance of Yahoo! stock should have anything to do with the weather in Montana! These arbitrary and completely unrelated variables were chosen intentionally for this example, to illustrate what it looks like when two sets of data are completely unrelated.

The above two examples are obviously not intended to provide a complete understanding of statistical correlation coefficient, but instead, to simply give you a frame of reference through which you can understand the correlation coefficients we will be talking about with regard to the Lyme-autism connection. There are many other aspects of correlation coefficient theory that were either simplified or not addressed in the examples. The important concept to keep in mind is that correlation coefficient ranges from 0 to 1, with 0 indicating no correlation at all, 1 indicating perfect correlation, and the range in between representing varying degrees of correlation. Generally, 0 to .1 means no correlation, .1 to .3 means a small correlation is present, .3 to .5 means there is a medium correlation, and .5 to 1 means that a strong correlation between the data exists.

Now let's shift gears from the example data sets to our Lyme-autism data sets. We will set out to compare Lyme disease statistics with autism statistics and see how strong the correlation is between the data. Is there a strong correlation between the incidences of Lyme disease and autism? A medium correlation? No correlation at all? Let's find out.

Chronological Correlation

First, we will look at the number of cases of both Lyme disease and autism reported by the CDC in the United States, without regard to geographical location, during the years 1993-2006. Below you can find the table with the raw data.

Year	Number of Cases of Lyme disease	Number of Cases of Autism
1993	8,257	19,058
1994	13,043	22,664
1995	11,700	29,076
1996	16,455	34,375
1997	12,801	42,517
1998	16,801	54,064
1999	16,273	66,043
2000	17,730	93,650
2001	17,029	114,841
2002	23,763	137,708
2003	21,273	163,773
2004	19,804	192,863
2005	23,305	224,293
2006	19,931	259,705

If you look at the data, it is clear that between 1993 and 2006, cases of both Lyme disease and autism were on the rise. But how similar is the pattern of increase? It is for this purpose that we turn to correlation coefficient. The correlation coefficient of the data is .80, indicating a strong correlation between the rising cases of Lyme disease and the rising cases of autism in the United States.

Although strong, this chronological correlation still leaves room for plenty of questions. Despite the fact that both diseases are on the rise, and that there exists a strong correlation coefficient which describes that rise, there may be entirely different causative factors in the increased prevalence of each disease. The fact that cases of each disease have exploded over the past decade or so does not mean that the diseases are necessarily connected. For example, the number of people who watch the Tour de France (the world's most popular bicycle race) on television has also exploded over the years 1993-2006. Does this mean that watching the Tour de France causes autism? Of course not! The same question must be asked of the Lyme-autism connection...is it a meaningful connection, or just a coincidental correlation?

To answer this question, we will again return to the idea repeated throughout this book: The Lyme-autism connection is not validated by each individual piece of the puzzle, but instead, by the *gestalt*—or *sum*—of the pieces. Additionally, the next statistical data set we will look at, that which compares geographical incidence of the two diseases, will provide further clarification. However, for the time being and for the purpose of discussion, let's address the above data as though the Lyme-autism connection were in fact valid.

You will note that the number of reported cases of autism throughout the United States is significantly greater than the number of reported cases of Lyme disease. Although both diseases started out with similar numbers in 1993 (8,257 cases of Lyme disease and 19,058 cases of autism), the two health conditions reached greatly divergent incidence as the years progressed, ending up with a spread of greater than 230,000 cases in 2006 (19,931 cases of Lyme disease and 259,705 cases of autism). Why the divergence? Why the exceedingly sharp rise in cases of autism, while cases of Lyme disease grew only gradually?

Assuming, for the sake of argument, that the Lyme-autism connection is in fact valid, the hypothesis which best explains this phenomenon is constructed from what we already know about the comparative accuracy in diagnosing the two conditions. Autism is typically diagnosed much more readily than is Lyme disease. It is likely that the real number of Lyme disease cases is actually rising much more rapidly than the statistics illustrate, even perhaps on a very similar course as autism. The question to ask is whether or not the actual number of Lyme disease cases is being accurately reported. Let's briefly look at some of the reasons why Lyme disease may be under-reported in comparison with autism.

For years now, numerous experts and scientific publications have been refuting the low CDC-reported Lyme disease statistics. In general, experts believe that the CDC grossly underestimates the true number of Lyme disease cases that occur each year. An example of a professional publication which questions the CDC's Lyme disease statistics is the *Townsend Letter for Doctors and Patients*, an alternative medicine journal published monthly. Edited by Jonathon Collin, MD, with numerous professional editorial advisors, including Dharma S. Khalsa, MD, and Robert Ronzio, Ph.D., this periodical reported in July, 2004, that the number of Lyme disease cases per year in the United States is close to 200,000—a much higher number than the CDC's reporting, which varies between 8,000 and 24,000 cases per year.

The Townsend Letter for Doctors and Patients agrees with the majority of research being published in modern times. It is generally agreed that official Lyme disease statistics are grossly under-represented, and that such under-representation occurs for three primary reasons: first, most U.S. physicians are not trained to look for the infection, so Lyme sufferers are often not tested for it; second, if the physicians are trained and the tests are given, the currently available laboratory tests often lead to false-negative results; and third, even in the event of positive Lyme disease test results, the CDC's "reporting criteria" only acknowledge a very narrow cross-section of positive test results as true cases of Lyme disease.

Additionally, as we have mentioned, the autism diagnosis is easier to make than the Lyme diagnosis due to the symptomology of the two diseases. While complex and not well understood, autism is not considered a difficult diagnosis—at least in comparison to Lyme disease. Because the symptoms of autism are typically more well-understood and recognized than the symptoms of Lyme disease, it is usually diagnosed fairly easily as a child grows up. The effects of Lyme disease, at least during adult onset, can be much more elusive and inconspicuous, leading to missed diagnoses. Lyme disease and autism are both elusive diseases, but Lyme disease is the more elusive of the two.

Autism has also received more political and mainstream attention than Lyme disease over the past several decades. This may have resulted in broader awareness among physicians, leading to more prompt and accurate diagnosis when compared with Lyme disease.

The correlation coefficient becomes much more interesting if we throw away the CDC Lyme disease statistics and substitute them with the more widely accepted recognition that Lyme disease is, in fact, under-reported. Although the precise numbers have not been accurately or thoroughly quantified at the time of this book's writing, several sources (including *The Townsend Letter for Doctors and Patients)* give estimations approximating an incidence of 200,000 cases of Lyme disease per year.

Using a linear interpolation model beginning with 8,257 cases of Lyme disease in 1993 (as reported by the CDC) and ending with 200,000 cases of Lyme disease in 2006 (as generally agreed upon by the Lyme disease clinicians, researchers and editorial advisors), the following table results:

Year	Number of Cases of Lyme disease	Number of Cases of Autism
1993	8,257	19,058
1994	15,978	22,664
1995	31,956	29,076
1996	47,934	34,375
1997	63,912	42,517
1998	79,890	54,064
1999	95,868	66,043
2000	111,846	93,650
2001	127,824	114,841
2002	143,802	137,708
2003	159,780	163,773
2004	175,758	192,863
2005	191,736	224,293
2006	200,000	259,705

The correlation coefficient of this hypothetical set of data is .96, indicating a very strong correlation. Granted, in this table, the cases of Lyme disease presented are only estimations, yet they are based on expert opinion and they represent what may be a more accurate picture than what the CDC purports as the incidence of Lyme disease.

The true correlation coefficient probably lies somewhere between .80 and .96. In any event, all of the possible correlation coefficients included in this range indicate a strong correlation between the incidence of Lyme disease and the incidence of autism between the years 1993 and 2006.

Let's now move on from looking at the chronological correlation between the two diseases to examine their geographical correlation.

Geographical Correlation

As we mentioned earlier, mere chronological correlation is not sufficient data upon which to build our argument and is relatively insignificant (think of the Tour de France example). It is for this reason that we will now seek to clarify the Lyme-autism relationship by introducing another set of data which examines the epidemiological statistics from a different perspective: the incidence of Lyme disease and autism as reported in 2006, categorized geographically for each state in the United States. If a correlation in this data also exists, then the Lyme-autism connection becomes considerably more plausible. If you find a high number of Lyme disease cases in the same states where you find a high number of autism cases, then we have just placed another piece in the Lyme-autism puzzle. The below findings have been roughly corroborated with the findings presented in the *Medical Hypothesis* journal article presented in Chapter 4.

Below you will find a table with the raw data, and following the table, you will see the information presented in a bar graph for easier visual assimilation.

State	Cases of Autism Per 100 Children During '06-'07 School Year*	Cases of Lyme disease Per 100,000 Population During 2006**
New Mexico	0.23	0.2
Mississippi	0.24	0.1
Louisiana	0.29	0
Iowa	0.29	3.3
Colorado	0.29	0
Montana	0.36	0.1
DC	0.37	10.7

Alabama	0.37	0.2
North Dakota	0.37	1.1
Tennessee	0.38	0.2
Kentucky	0.39	0.2
South Carolina	0.39	0.5
Kansas	0.39	0.1
Arkansas	0.43	0
Nebraska	0.43	0.6
West Virginia	0.43	1.5
Oklahoma	0.43	0
South Dakota	0.45	0.1
Wyoming	0.46	0.2
Alaska	0.47	0.4
Utah	0.50	0.2
Texas	0.50	0.1
Delaware	0.51	56.5
Illinois	0.52	0.9
Florida	0.53	0.2
Arizona	0.54	0.2
Hawaii	0.56	0
Idaho	0.58	0.5
Ohio	0.58	0.4
New York	0.59	23.1
Georgia	0.61	0.1
Missouri	0.61	0.1
North Carolina	0.61	0.4
Washington	0.62	0.1
New Hampshire	0.63	46.9
Vermont	0.63	16.8
Virginia	0.64	4.7
California	0.65	0.2
Michigan	0.67	0.5
Nevada	0.69	0.2
Maryland	0.70	22.2

Wisconsin	0.71	26.4
Massachusetts	0.74	22.2
Pennsylvania	0.75	26.1
Rhode Island	0.78	28.8
Connecticut	0.81	51
Indiana	0.86	0.4
New Jersey	0.87	27.9
Oregon	1.14	0.2
Maine	1.15	25.6
Minnesota	1.23	17.7

Sources:
*Thoughtful House Center for Children / Fighting Autism Foundation
**United States Centers for Disease Control (CDC)

This data is sorted from lowest to highest incidence of autism/state.

The above chart illustrates cases of Lyme disease per 100,000 people and cases of autism per 100 people. Why the large divergence in this common denominator? This question will be addressed in a few pages. The short answer is that cases of autism are reported more frequently than cases of Lyme disease.

The correlation coefficient for the geographical association between Lyme-disease and autism in the states which comprise the United States is .42, which is a medium correlation, and is only .08 away from being a strong correlation.

On the graph on the next page, note the distinct and unmistakable clumping of Lyme disease cases (black bars) in the states with the highest incidence of autism (gray bars). When the data is presented in bar graph format, this clumping is quite shocking. In general, the states with the highest incidence of Lyme disease are clearly the same states with the highest incidence of autism.

In comparison with chronological correlation, the medium-strength geographical correlation we have just seen is more

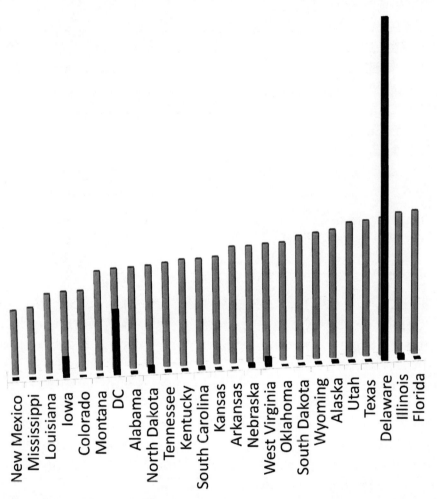

important and significant. This is because the chronological comparison (that is, the corollary rise in the number of cases of both diseases over the last 15 years) simply tells us that for some reason, both Lyme disease and autism are becoming more prevalent. This says nothing about whether or not they are related (again, think of the Tour de France example). Parallel but unrelated factors could be the cause of this similar rise. For example, Lyme disease cases may be increasing because of an increased tick population while autism cases may be on the rise due to new

■ — Cases of Lyme disease

▨ — Cases of autism

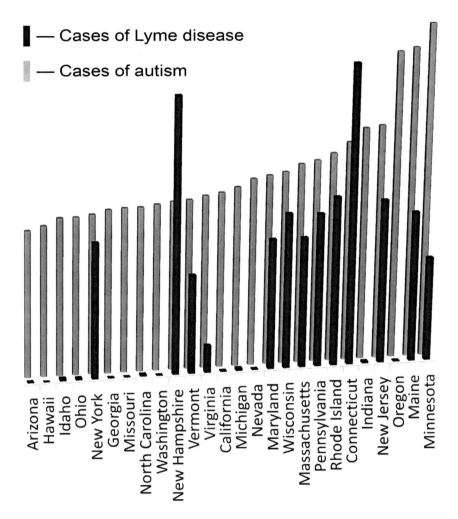

vaccination schedules. Obviously, the tick population has nothing to do with childhood vaccinations.

On the other hand, the geographical correlation between the two diseases is quite telling. To understand the reason for this, it is first necessary to understand the geographic nature of Lyme disease. Most diseases do not show higher or lower prevalence based on geography. For example, diabetes cases have nothing to do with where a person lives—instead, diabetes is strongly correlated with such non-geographical factors as genetics, diet, and obesity. In comparison, Lyme disease cases are highly concentrated in certain geographical locations, specifically, where tick populations are high, and even more specifically, where the high tick populations are infected with Lyme disease (some ticks do not carry the bacteria). This makes Lyme disease unique in that its prevalence is intimately connected with very specific, very distinctive, independent variables. We do not merely say that Lyme disease occurs in "warmer climates" or "wetter areas." No, we can go further and really isolate the offending variable: we can say with precise specificity that Lyme disease *is more prevalent in and only in areas where ticks thrive and are infected with Lyme bacteria.*

The story that begins to unfold, then, is that of a disease which has historically not been found to correlate with geographical factors (autism) becoming linked with a disease which is correlated with geographical factors (Lyme disease). Although the strength of the correlation is only "medium," it is statistically significant. And in this vein we are not merely saying that autism is more likely to occur in "warmer climates" or "wetter areas." Instead, because of what we know about the specificity of Lyme disease incidence (that it occurs in areas with high populations of infected ticks), we can be specific and distinctive in our conclusion about autism prevalence: that it is correlated with the specific condition of higher infected tick populations.

By now you can probably see the subtle, yet incredibly powerful insight we have into the correlation between the two diseases. At first, the seemingly simple and innocent geographical correlation might be dismissed as coincidence or the result of extraneous factors. However, when you look more closely, you can see that this correlation is far from innocent. It is very specific and meaningful and it tells us a great deal about a possible Lyme-autism connection.

Now, a disclaimer. Admittedly, the Lyme-autism connection is hypothetical at this point. It certainly is possible that there are variables which we are not recognizing or addressing. The geographical correlation between Lyme disease and autism is by no means proof that the correlation relationship is causative. When viewed independently from the rest of the information in this book, the geographical correlation between Lyme disease and autism does leave room for alternate explanations. However, when you add to the picture the many other arguments described in this book, such as similar symptoms, maternal transfer of the infection, and paralleling physiological disease processes, the case for a causal Lyme-autism connection gains more momentum. Remember, each puzzle piece is not sufficient to stand on its own, but when combined with other pieces, the completed puzzle is a lot more convincing.

We have now laid all of the puzzle pieces on the table for your thoughtful consideration. By no means has this book presented the whole picture; it will likely be years before such a picture exists. However, hopefully you have been challenged to think about Lyme disease and autism in a new light.

The final chapter will move away from presenting arguments for the Lyme-autism connection and instead provide practical guidance on how to get help if you or a loved one is dealing with a potential Lyme-autism diagnosis.

After Chapter 7, the Appendices will offer you supporting information, including mothers' stories, background data on Lyme disease, testing methodology, and other key reference materials.

Chapter 7
Getting Help

You've read it several times by now, but it is worth repeating and it is especially important in this chapter: because the Lyme-autism connection is still very new and undergoing initial research, diagnosis and treatment guidelines are far from complete. In fact, as you read this, the LIA Foundation is probably planning one of their annual conferences during which patients, parents, and practitioners from all around the country gather to roundtable about the Lyme-autism connection, hoping to gain much-needed insight into the diagnosis and treatment processes.

Instead of giving you guidelines for diagnosis and treatment, what this chapter will do is point you towards resources which will help you deal with a potential Lyme-autism diagnosis. Note that Appendix A provides various testing laboratories and methodologies which are currently being used to identify tick-borne infections and other problems in autistic children (as well as adults).

Of course, the first place you should visit for getting help is the LIA Foundation website: www.liafoundation.org. After you have spent some time on the website and signed up for the LIA Foundation email newsletter, your next step in the journey will be to locate a physician who can help you.

Finding a physician

In finding clinical help, the first order of business for you is to rendezvous with a licensed physician who is both Lyme-literate and autism-literate. Until recently, interdisciplinary expertise in these two conditions was virtually impossible to find in a health care practitioner. And, even as this book is being published, such physicians are still difficult to locate. However, as time passes, doctors are becoming increasingly aware of both Lyme disease and autism, and they are even beginning to acknowledge a possible connection between the two disorders. The publication of this book will hopefully accelerate the rate at which this awareness permeates modern medicine in America and throughout the world.

Although doctors have begun to recognize the Lyme-autism connection, no formal organization of Lyme-autism-literate doctors exists at the time of this book's publication. If such an organization were to be formed, it would obviously be the ideal resource through which to locate a Lyme-autism-literate doctor in your area. Frequently checking the LIA Foundation website at www.liafoundation.org will keep you apprised of the origination of such an organization.

In the meantime, there do exist independent associations of Lyme-literate physicians and autism-literate physicians from which you can get a physician referral. If you are unable to locate a physician versed in both diseases, the next best option is to make an appointment with either a Lyme-literate doctor or an autism-literate doctor. Assuming you find a physician versed in only one of the two diseases, you will need to take the initiative to educate him or her about the Lyme-autism connection. If visiting a Lyme physician, you will need to provide education on autism, and if visiting an autism physician, you will need to provide education on Lyme disease. Start by bringing a copy of this book to your physician and informing your physician about the LIA Foundation. You may end up deciding to retain the services of two doctors: one in the autism field and one in the Lyme disease field. If this is the approach you take, you should make sure that the two doctors are willing to collaborate with one another to develop a customized treatment plan.

Before directing you to the contact information for Lyme-literate and autism-literate doctors, a very important note:

Whatever you do, do not simply walk into any random general practitioner's office or general infectious disease doctor's office! Awareness of Lyme disease and/or autism is already very low among U.S. physicians—with the lowest level of awareness occurring in relation to Lyme disease. By seeing a doctor who is not versed in either of the two conditions, you are almost guaranteeing that you will be sent out of the office empty-handed, if not ridiculed. Presently, Lyme patients have a difficult time gaining recognition and validation in the United States. In fact, most U.S. physicians do not even acknowledge the existence of chronic Lyme disease (see Appendix B). When we are talking about Lyme disease and autism in the same patient, the chances of finding an educated physician decrease even further. You want to do everything you can to ensure that the odds are in your favor when selecting a physician. The first step toward placing the odds in your favor is to start with the most knowledgeable physician you can find instead of wasting time trying to educate other, potentially closed-minded doctors.

The one exception to the rule of finding an autism- and/or Lyme-literate physician at the outset is if you should happen to have a strong relationship with a general practitioner who is not aware of these two conditions but who has instead proven to you over past relationship that he or she is open-minded, accommodating, humble, and inquisitive. Such a physician (often a family friend, or, perhaps, a relative) may be able to help you by mere virtue of the fact that he or she may be willing to do what it takes to become educated on Lyme disease and autism. After all, when it comes to Lyme- and/or autism-literate physicians, the key qualities to seek are open-mindedness and humility.

However, if you approach this trusted doctor and they are hostile toward your hypothesis that you or your child may be suffering from Lyme disease and/or autism, then run the other way! There is no point in wasting your time trying to change a doctor's mind when you can instead spend your time and energy cultivating a professional relationship with one of the hundreds of physicians out there who will be accommodating and helpful to you. The simple fact is that most physicians are not only ignorant of the Lyme-autism connection, but they are actually taught in medical school to blindly dismiss suggestions from patients directing them to new areas of research. This type of dogma is ingrained in most physicians. Instead of fighting it, just accept that the Lyme-autism field is years ahead of its time, and find someone who is already on the right bus, so to speak.

The importance of finding a helpful, informed physician cannot be over-stated. Countless parents and patients have lost years of life, spent thousands of dollars, and endured immeasurable stress in hopeless arguments with closed-minded physicians, all the while unaware of the helpful and resourceful physician who may be practicing medicine just a few blocks down the road.

Also keep in mind that simply finding an autism-literate or Lyme-literate physician is not enough. Even finding one who is literate in both subjects is not enough. In addition to such litera-cy, a physician must also prove to you that he or she has an open mind and is willing to pursue ongoing education. The reason for this requirement is simply that both Lyme disease and autism are currently not well understood, and any physician who suc-cessfully cares for patients of these disorders must be committed to remaining on the cutting edge of modern medical science and interventions. This is especially difficult for physicians given their demanding work schedules and lack of time for keeping up with new research and ideas. You need to make sure your chosen doctor can dedicate the time it takes to not only become edu-cated, but also stay educated.

Additionally, make sure your physician knows that the Lyme-autism connection does not just involve Borrelia infection, but also dozens of other co-infections, including Babesia, Bartonella, Ehrlichia, mycoplasma, and many others. Or, if he or she does not already know this, make sure that he or she is open-minded enough to consider the possibility.

Finally (are you getting tired of all the requirements yet?), do not forget that *you*, as the patient (or patient's advocate) are ulti-mately responsible for your healthcare. Do not buy into the lie that you are a "consumer of prepackaged health care." Contrary to what the medical establishment would have you believe, there is no success to be found with blindly relying on the medical establishment. The responsibility for your success or failure in healing lies with no one other than you, and you alone! Do not cave in to the enticing desire for easy answers from a physician or specialist who seems to know it all. While it may feel comfort-able to blindly rely on decrees passed down by medical professionals, the truth is that such comfort is short-lived and the only real road to success requires your active questioning, participation, and intellectual engagement in the healing process.

With these many caveats out of the way, let's finally move on to the topic of actually finding an appropriate physician.

FINDING A LYME-LITERATE MEDICAL DOCTOR (LLMD)

Due to political controversy and legal challenges facing Lyme doctors, most of them prefer to keep a low profile. For this reason, they can be difficult to find. Additionally, good etiquette in the Lyme disease community dictates that when discussing doctors in public (including public internet discussion groups), their names should be kept private. If your doctor tells you that he or she is okay with his or her name being public, then you may be able to ignore this etiquette. However, when in doubt, assume that the above is true.

Getting a Lyme-literate physician referral:

1. **Lymenet.org "Seeking a Physician" Forum:** You can get a custom referral to an LLMD from www.lymenet.org. When you reach the homepage, click on "Flash Discussion," and then click on "Seeking a Doctor." You will be asked to provide your city, state, and contact information, and a Lymenet.org forum member will contact you with a physician referral.

2. **Lyme Disease Association Doctor Referral Service:** Visit www.lymediseaseassociation.org and click on "Doctor Referral." You will be asked for your contact information and a doctor referral will be provided.

3. **International Lyme and Associated Diseases Society (ILADS).** Contacting ILADS may also be helpful in your search for a physician. Use their website: www.ilads.org.

FINDING AN AUTISM-LITERATE MEDICAL DOCTOR

1. **Defeat Autism Now! (DAN) Doctors:** DAN is an organization which includes participating physicians who are educated in the treatment of autism. To find a DAN physician, visit www.autism.com and navigate to the DAN portion of the website. This website can be a bit cumbersome and there are many pages to navigate, however, the website does include a complete list of practitioners located both inside and outside of the United States.

2. **American College for Advancement in Medicine (ACAM) Doctors:** ACAM is a well-recognized organization focusing on alternative and integrative medicine. The physicians in the ACAM directory are generally regarded as forward-thinking, open-minded, excellent doctors. According to their website, ACAM's vision is to be "the voice of Integrative Medicine." These physicians may be helpful when dealing with Lyme disease and/or autism. To receive a referral to a physician in your area, visit www.acam.org and navigate to the "Physician Referral" portion of the website.

USING INTERNET DISCUSSION GROUPS TO LOCATE A PHYSICIAN

Another way to locate a physician is to visit one of the many free online discussion groups related to Lyme disease and/or autism, and simply post a message requesting that forum participants who live in your geographical area send you a private email with information about their health care practitioner. Remember to request that this information be transmitted *privately* to respect the privacy of health care practitioners. The advantage of this method for locating a physician is that the recommendation you receive will more than likely be backed by personal experience from the person telling you about the doctor. In other words, in addition to finding a doctor in your geographical area, you will probably also find a doctor who is proficient, professional, and worthy of recommendation.

Brief Tips for Formulating a Treatment Plan

While this book will not provide a treatment plan for you, it will offer some general tips.

First, beware of one-size-fits-all treatment plans. One-size-fits-all treatment plans are not only ineffective, but they can also be dangerous because one person's cure may be another person's poison (due to the huge variances in our individual biochemistries). You and your doctor must step out into the highly individualized adventure of applying knowledge of your situation, analytical skills, and trial and error to the process of building a treatment program. Your trusted physician(s) are your allies during this process not only because they are educated and licensed to practice medicine, but also because they will (or should, at least) provide you with the one-on-one attention necessary to understand your unique and special circumstances.

To formulate a unique treatment plan for the patient in question, you will need to make use of all available resources. The following is an approximate list of the steps you should take:

1. Take the information in this book to your physician, who should already have a solid education in Lyme disease and/or autism treatment. If your physician is Lyme-literate, help him or her to become autism-literate, and vice versa.

2. You and your physician should dialogue about the unique health challenges facing the patient. Tests should be ordered and a clinical evaluation conducted. Your physician should not

just rely on standard laboratory tests, but he/she should also have knowledge of some of the more cutting edge Lyme disease tests available (see Appendix A).

3. You and your physician should discuss the LIA Foundation, attend their annual conference if possible, and stay up-to-date on their latest research. It would be very beneficial for you to purchase the LIA Foundation conference DVDs available from www.lymebook.com/autism and loan them to your physician.

4. You should combine your special knowledge of your child (or the patient, whomever he or she may be) with your physician's special approach to formulating a treatment plan. The treatment strategy should be based on a foundation which includes the combination of a parent or patient's experience, instinct, and knowledge with a Lyme- and/or autism-literate physician's education, experience and instinct.

5. You and your physician must remain flexible, adaptable, and willing to alter the program as additional information becomes available in the research field and you observe the patient's response to the treatment program.

6. Your physician should remain committed to a close, one-on-one relationship with the patient and/or caretaker. You should expect this relationship to continue for months or years.

Treatment Resources

Below you will find additional resources that will point you to external sources of information that can help you learn more about available treatments. This section of information focuses on Lyme disease, not autism.

When researching treatment options, remember to make your first stop the LIA Foundation website: www.liafoundation.org. Because the LIA Foundation specifically focuses on the *connec-*

tion between the two diseases, their information, provided by physicians, researchers and parents, will be more useful than information which focuses on Lyme disease or autism separately.

WEBSITES

External websites not affiliated with Bryan Rosner or BioMed Publishing Group:

1. www.ilads.org: International Lyme and Associated Diseases Society. This website contains treatment guidelines written by Dr. Joseph Burrascano, one of the nation's leading Lyme doctors. These treatment guidelines are considered by the majority of Lyme disease doctors and researchers to be the gold standard for long-term care. This website should be one of your first stops.

2. www.lymediseaseassociation.com: This is one of the largest and most politically active Lyme disease associations in the United States. The Lyme Disease Association hosts conferences and provides literature to physicians and patients. They are also responsible, in part, for helping to open the Lyme disease Research Center (www.columbia-lyme.org) at Columbia University. Also offered is a physician referral service through which you can locate a Lyme Literate Medical Doctor (LLMD) in your area.

3. www.lymenet.org: This is the world's largest online support group for Lyme disease sufferers, with over 10,000 members. Here you can communicate with other Lyme sufferers and also read about the latest antibiotic treatment guidelines. Also offered is a physician referral service through which you can locate a Lyme Literate Medical Doctor (LLMD) in your area.

Websites hosted by Bryan Rosner and/or BioMed Publishing Group:

1. www.lymebook.com/autism: Source to purchase DVDs from past Lyme-Autism Connection conferences.

2. www.defeatlyme.com: On this website, which hosts another book I wrote, entitled *The Top 10 Lyme Disease Treatments,* numerous free excerpts are available to read online. One of these excerpts is entitled "Non-pharmaceutical (Natural) Antibiotics for Lyme disease." In this excerpt, you can read about numerous herbal and natural antibiotics, and also find the contact information for the manufacturers, retailers, and distributors of these products. Additionally, one of the other excerpts available free of charge online is entitled "Three Forms of Borrelia burgdorferi," and includes a chart which briefly discusses various antibiotic choices for each form of the bacteria. Yet another excerpt describes sauna therapy as it is used to provide detoxification during Lyme disease treatment.

3. www.lymebook.com/articlelibrary: The article library offered by BioMed Publishing Group contains several useful articles for learning more about the topics discussed in this chapter. The articles include the following titles:

   a. *Sample Lyme Disease Treatment Plan—Calendar, Chart, and Discussion*

   b. *Four Immune-Supporting Supplements Every Lyme Disease Sufferer Needs to Know About—And Where to Buy Them*

   c. *Homeopathy and Lyme disease*

   d. *Everything You Always Wanted to Know About the CD-57 Test—But Were too Sick to Ask*

4. www.lymebook.com/resources: This is the internet repository for website links maintained by Bryan Rosner and BioMed Publishing Group. Here you will find links to numerous resources.

5. www.lymevideoblog.com: Bryan Rosner's video blog, in which you can watch Bryan discuss numerous important Lyme-related topics.

6. www.lymebook.com/newsletter: Sign up for Bryan Rosner's newsletter and be kept up-to-date on current findings.

7. www.lymecommunity.com: Internet discussion forum offering free membership. Established for the purpose of communication and collaboration among Lyme disease sufferers.

8. www.lymebook.com: Selection of related books and DVDs.

BOOKS

1. *The Lyme Disease Solution,* by Kenneth Singleton, MD. Dr. Singleton is one of the first physicians ever to write a book on the diagnosis and treatment of Lyme disease. This book includes a great deal of information on antibiotic use, both pharmaceutical and non-pharmaceutical. A must-read for anyone dealing with Lyme disease.
Available from www.lymebook.com/lyme-disease-solution.

2. *The Top 10 Lyme Disease Treatments,* by Bryan Rosner. This was the second book I wrote on Lyme disease.
Available from www.defeatlyme.com.

3. *The 2008 Lyme Disease Annual Report,* by Bryan Rosner. This book serves as Bryan Rosner's annual newsletter and offers updates on treatments, political issues, and other relevant topics. If you purchase the report direct from the publisher, it includes a free download of Bryan Rosner's 9-page e-article

entitled *Four Immune-Supporting Supplements Every Lyme disease Sufferer Needs to Know About—And Where to Buy Them.*
Available from www.lymebook.com.

4. *Healing Lyme*, by Stephen Harrod Buhner. Published in 2004, and written by a master herbalist, this book provides detailed information on specific herbal remedies which target various aspects of the Lyme disease complex, including specific options for non-pharmaceutical antibiotic therapy. Also a must-read.
Available from www.amazon.com.

5. Dr. James Schaller (www.personalconsult.com) has also released numerous very helpful books, including *The Diagnosis and Treatment of Babesia, The Diagnosis and Treatment of Bartonella,* and *Mold Illness and Mold Remediation Made Simple.* According to Dr. Schaller, addressing Babesia, Bartonella, and mold problems can have a tremendous positive impact on the healing process.
Dr. Schaller's books are available from www.lymebook.com.

Closing Argument

The purpose of this book is not to convince you of the validity of the Lyme-autism connection. The connection is not yet proven. However, in the battle for our children's health, the best weapon we have is information. If we did our job in writing this book, you should come away from reading it with the information you need to conduct additional research and come to your own conclusions. Our job was to equip you with the facts and current data.

Let's briefly review several of the key points covered in this book.

1. Autism involves the immune system, and many of the immune dysfunctions seen in autism are the same as those seen in Lyme disease.

2. Numerous infections appear to be involved in autism, one of which is Borrelia burgdorferi (the Lyme disease bacteria). Borrelia appears to be one of the more important infections due to its skyrocketing prevalence and epidemic proportions.

3. The Lyme-autism connection has been substantiated by clinical experience, both in the physician's office and at home among numerous mothers.

4. Borrelia can be transmitted from mother to baby during pregnancy, resulting in early childhood infection.

5. The symptoms of Lyme disease overlap with the symptoms of autism, and in fact, the two diseases have in common many of the same "mimicking diagnoses." Both Lyme disease and autism are characterized by clustering of these diseases within family histories.

6. The Lyme-autism connection is being studied with increasing frequency, by researchers with an ever-growing list of qualifications and credentials.

7. The connection is supported by geographical, chronological, and statistical analysis of the epidemiology of the two diseases, with strong and medium correlation coefficients, respectively.

8. The Lyme-autism connection is comprised of not one or two elements, but instead, numerous puzzle pieces which support one another to create and substantiate the connection hypothesis.

9. If you intend to take action and apply Lyme disease treatment to your child, please do so only under the supervision of a licensed physician.

10. This field is evolving rapidly. To stay up to date, keep connected with the LIA Foundation, www.liafoundation.org.

Additionally, sign up for Bryan's email newsletter at www.lymebook.com/newsletter.

We leave you now with a challenge. We challenge you to use your mind and your analytical skills to formulate your own opinion about the Lyme-autism connection. Furthermore, whether you become convinced of the connection or not, we challenge you to roll up your sleeves, become a detective, and get to the bottom of your child's health problems. Commit to staying up to date with the latest research and findings, to ensure that you are well equipped to provide the best care possible for your child. Do not rely solely on your physician. As a parent, you must be empowered to do what is necessary.

Your situation, your child, and the health of your family are unique. The only person well-suited to make decisions for you, is you. Make these decisions with confidence, knowing that if you are too fearful to make decisions, someone else will make them for you, and they will certainly make decisions inferior to those which you are capable of.

The most important realization we want you to walk away with is that autism is a physical disorder, not a psychological disorder. Psychological disorders leave caretakers hopeless as these disorders are mysterious and untreatable. Physical disorders, on the other hand, can be dealt with by using rational, measured, scientific treatments. There is something physically wrong in the bodies of autistic children. Therefore, physical interventions can be successful. Your child's condition is treatable. We may not have all the answers about *how* to treat autism, but we are beginning the quest from a place of hope, not despair.

Our best wishes go out to you and we deeply desire that your family would experience speedy, permanent healing.

Appendices

APPENDIX A
TESTING FOR LYME DISEASE AND CO-INFECTIONS

As you know from reading this book (and will learn more about in Appendix B) Lyme disease diagnosis and treatment is highly controversial and difficult. Unfortunately, there is not a general consensus on which types of tests are most accurate and useful for diagnosing Lyme disease. Numerous tests are available, each of which uses different methodology for detecting Borrelia and related co-infections.

What is agreed on, however, is that most Lyme disease tests can produce false-negative test results (meaning that the test indicates no presence of the Lyme infection when, in fact, it is present). For this reason, regardless of which test(s) you choose, it is critical to keep in mind that a negative result does not mean that Lyme disease is not present!

Robert Bransfield, MD, (www.mentalhealthandillness.com) offers 27 reasons why Lyme disease tests produce false-negative results:

1. Recent infection before immune response

2. Antibodies are in immune complexes

3. Spirochete encapsulated by host tissue (i.e.: lymphocytic cell walls)

4. Spirochete is deep in host tissue (i.e.: fibroblasts, neurons, etc.)

5. Blebs in body fluid, no whole organisms needed for PCR

6. No spirochetes in body fluid on day of test

7. Genetic heterogeneity (300 strains, 100 in U.S.)

8. Antigenic variability

9. Surface antigens change with temperature

10. Utilization of host protease instead of microbial protease

11. Spirochete in dormancy phase (L-form) with no cell walls

12. Recent antibiotic treatment

13. Recent anti-inflammatory treatment

14. Concomitant infection with Babesia may cause immunosuppression

15. Other causes of immunosuppression

16. Lab with poor technical capability for Lyme disease

17. Lab tests not standardized for late stage disease

18. Lab tests labeled "for investigational use only"

19. CDC criteria is epidemiological, not a diagnostic criteria

20. Lack of standardized control

21. Most controls use only a few strains as reference point

22. Few organisms are sometimes present

23. Encapsulated by glycoprotein "S-layer" which impairs immune recognition

24. "S"- layer binds to IgM

25. Immune deficiency

26. Possible down regulation of immune system by cytokines

27. Revised W.B. criteria fails to include most significant antigens

In the event that a negative test result is received, there are other methods by which the presence of Lyme disease can be confirmed. One such method is known as a "therapeutic trial," in which a person who is suspected of having Lyme disease undergoes a trial period of Lyme disease therapy for the purpose of determining whether or not the therapy leads to clinical improvement. If clinical improvement or herxheimer reactions result, there is a high probability that, despite negative test results, Lyme disease is actually present.

Another method for confirming or denying the presence of Lyme disease after a negative test result is to simply use a different testing method. The following section includes general information about the available testing methodology. The Lyme Induced Autism (LIA) Foundation provided significant contribution to this section via their handout entitled *Testing for Lyme/Borrelia and Multiple-Infections.*

In addition to testing for Lyme disease and co-infections, it is also helpful to identify which heavy metals, if any, are present. See Appendix C for more information on testing for and treating heavy metal toxicity.

Testing Guidelines for Infections and Parasites

Testing for Lyme disease, Borreliosis and multiple-infections can be difficult to understand. We hope that this guide will help to narrow down the lab testing and options available. One thing to keep in mind is that many times the lab testing that our insurance generally pays for is not necessarily the most appropriate or accurate available. To avoid needless blood draws, wasted time and resources, we recommend getting the appropriate testing done first so that parents can have a clear picture of their child's infection load prior to starting therapy interventions.

Testing for Lyme disease (Borrelia burgdorferi), Babesia, Anaplasma, Ehrlichia and Bartonella

Testing for Lyme disease/Borrelia and other infections is not a simple task. A person with a compromised immune system may not make the necessary antibodies needed to generate an accurate reading. No test is perfect and someone may have the organism(s) in their body and still have a negative test result. A positive antibody test shows evidence of the body's response to an organism, not the organism itself.

There may also be multiple strains of an organism, yet we typically can only test for one, such as Bartonella, which has nine pathogenic strains but antibody tests only exist for one or two. Therefore, testing should be viewed as helpful information that must be considered within the context of the patient's history and physical findings—testing should not be considered 100% accurate for a final diagnosis.

The "lyme titer" or "ELISA" test that is often first ordered as a "screen" by some clinicians can be very inaccurate. The Lyme/Borrelia "Western Blot" is a more sensitive test. Standard laboratories do not test for all of the "bands" in the Western Blot that are specific to Lyme/Borrelia. Many people will get a false negative from the commercial labs or from a doctor who is not trained to interpret tests properly. It is important to note that if the test comes back negative, the results may be inaccurate.

Testing Laboratories

Although the LIA Foundation does not recommend a specific lab, the following is a list of labs which we believe offer a superior quality of test compared to the standard lab.

IGeneX
This lab has a variety of panels and individual tests available. Most Lyme literate practitioners will order the Western Blot IgG / IgM for Borrelia (#188, #189). This Western Blot is the only one that tests for every Borrelia-specific band. They may also choose to order the PCR or IFA as well. IGeneX also offers testing for Babesia, Ehrlichia, Anaplasma and Bartonella (in addition to antibody tests for these infections, you should also strongly consider the "FISH" test [discussed below], which is a direct fluorescent staining of the organism). IGeneX offers a "complete co-infection panel"(#5090) and also a "western regional complete co-infection panel" (#5080). A PCR test is best done during a symptom "flare" or during menses, if applicable. IGeneX recommends having at least two Borrelia specific bands, in addition to associated symptoms, to make a positive diagnosis.

Phone: (800) 832-3200
Website: www.igenex.com

NeuroScience/NeuroImmunology Labs
This lab has 3 panels which include the standard Western Blot, antibody testing, and testing for many of the co-infections such as Babesia, Ehrlichia and Bartonella. Not all specific bands are checked on the Western Blot, only those in the CDC "panels." In addition, this lab does specialty testing for Autism Spectrum Disorder.

Phone: (715) 294-2852 - Email: info@neuroimmunologylabs.com

Central Florida Research

This lab offers a test called the Lyme Antigen Test by Flow Cytometry. Antigen tests detect the organism itself and, unlike antibody tests, antigen tests do not depend on the immune system's ability to produce pathogen-specific antibodies. This means that, in some cases, antigen tests may be more accurate than antibody tests.

Phone: (863) 956-3538
Website: www.centralfloridaresearch.com

Fry Clinical Labs

This lab does direct visual microscopy of a blood sample and thus can identify Babesia, Bartonella and others even when antibodies are not present or at very low levels. A positive visual identification of the pathogen(s) may be definitive; however, a result indicating that "no organisms were seen" does not necessarily rule out the possibility that the organisms are present but missed during the test. Some organisms, especially Lyme/Borrelia, are often difficult to detect due to their elusive presence in deep tissue which are not examined or visible during blood tests.

Phone: (480) 991-4555

Testing for Mycoplasma

According to research done by the Institute for Molecular Medicine and reported on their website at www.immed.org, "we have identified systemic infections, such as those produced by *Mycoplasma* species, *Chlamydia pneumoniae* and Human Herpes Virus-6 (HHV-6), in a high percentage of Autism Spectrum Disorder (ASD) patients, and these infections are likely to be important in determining the treatment strategies for many ASD patients."

Medical Diagnostic Laboratories (MDL)

Professor Garth Nicolson's work from the Institute for Molecular Medicine found that 58% of ASD children have multiple strains of Mycoplasma. This lab offers the "Mycoplasma General PCR test" and "Mycoplasma Fermentans PCR test." Also, HHV-6 (human herpes virus-6), can be tested here; both antibody and PCR.

Phone: (877) 269-0090
Website: www.mdlab.com

Testing for Viruses

It is a good idea to test for HHV-6 as many children have a significant viral load. A subset of children with autism have shown improvement by using anti-viral treatments.

ViraCor Laboratories

Direct effects of HHV-6 include fever, rash, hepatitis, encephalitis, pneumonitis and delay or suppression of bone marrow engraftment. This lab tests for HHV-6 by the PCR method.

Phone: (800) 305-5198
Website: www.viracor.com

Parasites, Yeast and Gastrointestinal Testing

The bodies of children and adults suffering from chronic illnesses are typically ideal environments for parasites and yeast. It is important to discover which microbes are causing trouble. Below is a list of labs which are commonly used for this type of testing.

Diagnos-Techs, Inc.

The "GI Health" and "Expanded GI Health" panels test for several types of parasites, food intolerances, gut function and general GI health.

Phone: (800) 878-3787
Website: www.diagnostechs.com

Genova Diagnostics

This lab offers several panels, including the "Parasitology profile" or, for a more detailed panel, the "Comprehensive Stool Analysis."

Phone: (800) 522-4762
Website: www.gdx.net

Great Plains Laboratory

Many physicians have confidence in this lab due to their specialized testing. For Candida testing, an "Organic Acid Test" or "Microbial OAT Panel" can give a clear picture as to the yeast or bacterial overgrowth in the patient.

Phone: (800) 288-0383
Website: www.greatplainslaboratory.com

Metametrix Clinical Laboratory

This laboratory can be used for stool cultures, organic acids, and metabolites of bacteria and pathogenic yeast. They also offer tests for fatty acids, metabolism, Krebs cycle issues, and functional vitamin deficiencies.

Phone: (800) 221-4640
Website: www.metametrix.com

Doctors Data

Doctors Data offers comprehensive stool analysis, parasitology, and microbiology panels which help to investigate the health of the GI tract. In addition, this lab is great for heavy metal toxicity testing.

Phone: (800) 323-2784
Website: www.doctorsdata.com

Heavy Metal Testing

It is well known that autism can be associated with heavy metal poisoning, by elements such as arsenic, copper, mercury, and others. For this reason, heavy metal testing should be conducted. The labs most often relied on are *Great Plains Laboratory* and *Doctors Data*. See Appendix C for more information. Since heavy metals are not always found in the blood and many prefer tissue, bone or other locations, this is a useful screen test. At times, it requires some expertise to read the results since some minerals can be high or low and either can be a flag for further follow up.

According to Dr. James Schaller, MD:

> *Based on my research, all Americans have levels of some toxic heavy metals which undermine optimal health. This research was based on using a wide variety of respected chelation challenge agents, and doing pre- and post- testing which fit each agent's mechanism. All patients were found to have heavy metal ranges that would undermine health.*
>
> *If this is true, why allow autistic or Lyme infected children to have this additional burden on neurologic and immune function to exist? There are many child-friendly chelation agents available at this time. So talk to an expert in chelation and read widely.*
>
> *Some health care professionals might be too frozen into using a limited number of options, and may not be familiar with the full range of non-IV options presently available.*

APPENDIX B
INTRODUCTION TO LYME DISEASE

This appendix contains an excerpt from my recently published book, The Top 10 Lyme Disease Treatments (available from www.lymebook.com). This excerpt is an introduction to Lyme disease. Please note that the discussion of Lyme disease treatment included in this excerpt was written with adult patients in mind, not children. Childhood Lyme disease requires different treatment approaches than adult Lyme disease. See Chapter 7 for more information on developing a treatment plan for children.

Welcome to the World of Lyme Disease

Lyme disease is a bacterial infection caused by Borrelia burgdorferi, an elongated, spiral-shaped bacteria transmitted to humans through the bite of a tick. Known as spirochetes, these bacteria are unusual, not well studied, elusive, difficult to cultivate in the laboratory and capable of advanced survival activities more commonly found in larger, more intelligent organisms.

Most Lyme disease literature erroneously reports that Lyme disease was first documented in Lyme, Connecticut, in the late 1970s. Actually, record of the infection dates back to 1883 when a German physician named Alfred Buchwald observed a degenerative skin condition which is presently hypothesized to have been a Lyme-related ailment. Subsequently in the United States, as early as 1920, physicians began correlating what are now known to be Lyme disease symptoms with tick bites. By 1950, doctors had already discovered that antibiotic therapy provided relief for the symptoms in question. Although it was not until the 1970s that the disease got its name, evidence from various sources makes it apparent that Lyme disease is much older than popularly believed.

First, the good news—in many cases of acute, recently acquired Lyme disease, pharmaceutical antibiotics (the standard treatment of choice) are effective in completely eradicating the infection or at least, permanently alleviating symptoms. Someone who goes hiking or camping, gets bitten by a tick, and rushes to their doctor with a bull's-eye rash and flu-like symptoms has a chance of getting completely cured. The generally accepted rule is that if antibiotic therapy can be initiated within 24 hours of a tick bite, Lyme disease is preventable.

Now, the bad news—there are dozens of reasons why it doesn't always happen this way. Unfortunately, the current mainstream medical procedures for diagnosing and treating Lyme disease can fail at many points in the diagnosis and treatment process, leading to prolonged suffering and frustration. The odds are stacked high against people suffering from Lyme disease. First we will examine obstacles in diagnosing Lyme disease and then we will look at problems with current treatment practices.

Obstacles in Diagnosis

Despite the vast and increasing prevalence of Lyme disease in the United States and other countries, many doctors are still not trained to look for the disease. Lack of training results from the misguided belief among mainstream medical colleges that Lyme disease is actually not a prevalent, rapidly spreading infection but instead, a rare and uncommon condition.

Some doctors will tell a sick person returning from a camping trip to take some Pepto-Bismol after diagnosing them with food poisoning from camping food. Other doctors will suggest Giardia, as a result of drinking contaminated stream water, and proclaim that the telltale bull's-eye rash is just a harmless insect bite or an allergic reaction to some grass or pollen or other irritant found in nature. Still other doctors will recommend watching symptoms for a few weeks to see if they improve on their own, after which time, if a person really had contracted Lyme disease, antibiotic therapy would be too late anyway. If the bacteria are allowed to survive in the body unchallenged by antibiotic therapy for more than a couple days, treatment becomes much more complicated and protracted because the bacteria invade and colonize many organs and tissues. For this reason, early detection and treatment are critical—yet they often do not occur because Lyme disease is not on the forefront of most physicians' minds.

If a physician is actually trained to look for Lyme disease and he/she orders a Lyme disease test, the next obstacle in the way of accurate diagnosis is the high probability of inaccurate, false-negative test results. As many as 60% of people infected with Lyme disease will actually produce a negative test result! This can happen because the antigens and antibodies which the tests look for are not present (or at least not detectable) in the body during a large part of the bacterial life cycle. Therefore, anyone who receives a negative Lyme disease test result in the presence of clinical symptoms should be suspicious and consider a therapeutic trial of Lyme disease therapy, a procedure in which a person suspecting Lyme disease is given a course of Lyme disease treatment to see if clinical improvement results.

An additional problem with laboratory tests is the processing period. Because processing a Lyme disease test can take a couple weeks, even if a positive result is received, it may be too late for antibiotic therapy to eradicate the infection.

Timing of symptom onset also contributes to missed diagnoses, even when dealing with a competent physician. Since symptoms often do not appear until several weeks or months after the infection is acquired, a person coming down with a mystery illness may not suspect Lyme disease even if they vaguely remembered a tick bite, because there may be no apparent association between the tick bite and the new symptoms. This confusion makes it difficult for even a good physician to sort out what is going on.

To make matters worse, in many cases, symptoms of Lyme disease may be delayed even longer than weeks or months. In some cases, symptoms may not appear until years after initial infection, leading to an even smaller probability of proper diagnosis. In addition, initial symptoms can be so subtle as to be mistaken for "growing pains" or "being out of shape". In these cases, tests would not even be ordered unless a shrewd physician or patient pieced together the puzzle. And, even if tests were ordered, the looming risk of a false-negative result creates more confusion.

New evidence has also identified other possible routes of transmission for the infection, including mother to child during pregnancy or breast-feeding, mosquito to human, and sexual intercourse. These routes of transmission are not recognized or acknowledged by most of mainstream medicine. This denial is in the face of glaring evidence to the contrary and is a cause for additional confusion when diagnosing Lyme disease. Because some Lyme disease sufferers have never spent much time outdoors, they will automatically be disqualified from Lyme disease screening—even if, in reality, they are subject to other risk factors such as a mother with Lyme disease.

Adding to the already stacked odds that a Lyme disease sufferer will not be diagnosed properly is the elusive and variable nature of the disease presentation itself. Lyme disease can and does manifest as dozens of different diseases and conditions which are conventionally believed to be incurable and unrelated to Borrelia burgdorferi infection. Examples of such diseases include Parkinson's, ALS, depression, arthritis, chronic fatigue syndrome, fibromyalgia, Epstein-Barr virus, candida, schizophrenia, multiple sclerosis, obsessive-compulsive disorder, and others. Because of its ability to mimic so many seemingly unrelated conditions, Lyme disease is known as the "great imitator." The ability for the disease to manifest in so many ways is a result of the spirochetes' capability of infecting each and every major organ system in the body. Unfortunately, most physicians do not suspect Lyme disease when dealing with one of these other conditions even though, in a significant number of cases, Lyme disease is the root cause.

As if the situation weren't bad enough already, many doctors do not acknowledge that Lyme disease exists in more than a few isolated parts of the United States. Chances are a person with a newly acquired Lyme disease infection will encounter a physician who does not believe the disease is native to the area in which they live. In reality, Lyme disease has been documented in every state in the United States and many countries throughout the world.

As you can see, diagnosing Lyme disease is a complicated task. Having awareness of this complexity is the first step toward healing those suffering from this affliction and toward ensuring that future diagnostic procedures become more reliable.

Obstacles in Treatment

The diagnosis process is unfortunately not the end of the obstacle field confronting Lyme disease sufferers. Even if diagnosed early and accurately, a Lyme disease sufferer faces sizable challenges in the treatment process.

Current antibiotic guidelines set forth by the Centers for Disease Control are vastly inadequate and based on antiquated, inaccurate, and unreliable data. While some people do get well by following these guidelines, a significant percentage do not. Many people remain sick despite a two or three week course of doxycycline or penicillin—the length and choice of antibiotic therapy which the Centers for Disease Control dogmatically and ignorantly insist is adequate treatment. Recent estimates suggest that up to 30% of Lyme disease cases do not get resolved after following these CDC guidelines.

A preponderance of research establishing the necessity of extended courses of antibiotic therapy for the unlucky 30% has been completely ignored by medical regulatory agencies. As a result, symptoms and misery can continue for the unlucky 30% even though the "right treatment" was given. People who are still infected despite antibiotic therapy have what is referred to as chronic Lyme disease. The chronic form of the disease is becoming an epidemic in the United States and abroad.

Or is it? A significant percentage of doctors and regulatory agencies do not recognize the existence of chronic Lyme disease. The prevailing belief is that if someone has Lyme disease and is treated with a several-weeklong course of antibiotics, they must, by definition, be cured. This belief fails to take into account the last 20 years of scientific research, as there have been numerous studies which demonstrate that Lyme disease bacteria are often still present in the body even after antibiotic therapy. In fact, some studies show that common antibiotic regimens have very little effect on the bacterial infection.

Doctors and researchers who do not acknowledge chronic Lyme disease have invented a bogus label for people who still have symptoms after a short course of antibiotics: "Post-Lyme Syndrome." Patients abused with this diagnosis are either told that nonliving bacterial toxins are keeping them ill, or worse, that remaining symptoms are psychiatric in nature and they should see a shrink who treats hypochondria and paranoia. So, many patients end up attempting to treat a raging bacterial infection with talk therapy. The truth is that chronic Lyme disease is in fact a real condition, caused by an active bacterial infection, and largely disparaged by conventional medicine.

The conclusion that chronic Lyme disease is not a valid medical condition is so preposterous, so irrational, so unscientific that one can't help but question whether the presiding research organizations are actually pursuing truth or instead, acting as puppets beholden to a political or medical agenda. There is simply too much research to ignore. And as time goes on, instead of behaving rationally and slowly examining new research and moving toward adoption of chronic Lyme disease as a real condition, the regulatory agencies seem to be going in the opposite direction and becoming more adamant about their erroneous conclusions.

The doctors who recognize chronic Lyme disease, and are willing to treat it, are few and far between. LLMDs use extended courses of very powerful antibiotics, sometimes in combinations of two or three drugs simultaneously, at much higher than FDA-approved dosages, to try to help people with chronic Lyme disease. Doctors who treat chronic Lyme disease are heroes with good intentions, coming to the rescue when no one else will.

But even if patient and LLMD are able to connect, there are still additional obstacles. Unfortunately, LLMDs who do step out on a limb and actually try to help people with chronic Lyme disease by reading the literature and implementing rational treatments are often persecuted, sued, disciplined by state medical boards, ridiculed, and at risk of losing their medical practice, as we have discussed in the previous section of the book. Increasing persecution and legal danger has led to the decision by many doctors not to treat Lyme disease patients, or at least, to adhere to the inadequate treatment guidelines established by the government.

Although it is becoming increasingly perilous, many LLMDs are willing to brave the legal climate because some people with chronic Lyme disease do recover by using extended courses of antibiotic therapy. In these cases, people who would have otherwise not recovered at all owe their lives to LLMDs. Offering hope to hopeless patients is the daily business of a Lyme disease doctor.

Unfortunately, there are some very significant drawbacks to long-term antibiotic therapy. Patients receiving long-term antibiotic therapy often face grueling battles with insurance companies as a result of skyrocketing medical bills. Because official government standards indicate that only a short course of antibiotics is necessary in the treatment of Lyme disease, many people are not able to get their extended treatment covered.

Another significant drawback to long-term antibiotic therapy is side effects. Because antibiotics are given in very high doses for long periods of time, side effects can be devastating. In some cases, the side effects can be worse than the disease. Many people end up with permanent damage to various organs caused by extended-course, high-dose antibiotic therapy.

The most significant drawback to long-term antibiotic therapy, though, is that it does not always work. The best antibiotics, given at high doses for months on end, often fail to eradicate the elusive and survival-oriented Lyme disease bacteria. In these cases, symptom improvement can be fragile and relapses are common. "Open-ended" antibiotic therapy is frequently required to keep some people stable. My first book, Lyme Disease and Rife Machines, has an in-depth explanation of exactly how and why antibiotics can fail.

The above treatment obstacles do not just exist in theory. The reality is that there are thousands of chronic Lyme sufferers who continuously live a miserable existence despite having attempted to get help from dozens of doctors.

As you can see, the situation can be quite hopeless. Lyme disease sufferers are left to try to find answers on their own between doctors' appointments where they are given anything from a diagnosis of paranoia to an inadequate course of antibiotics to a denial of insurance coverage. At every step in the diagnosis and treatment process, Lyme disease sufferers encounter an uphill battle which often leads to prolonged sickness, financial ruin, and unimaginable stress. Many Lyme disease sufferers live their lives in complete despair, having tried every antibiotic under the sun without lasting relief.

The bottom line on diagnosing and treating Lyme disease is that there are many ways to end up with the infection but not many ways to get rid of it. *[End Excerpt. The book from which this excerpt was taken can be purchased at www.lymebook.com].*

APPENDIX C
TESTING FOR AND TREATING HEAVY METAL POISONING

In modern times, it is well known that heavy metals such as mercury, lead, and arsenic lead to a wide array of neurological disorders in adults and children, and can contribute to the onset and severity of autism. This topic has received an explosive amount of attention over the past 10 years, and dozens of books, hundreds of websites, and countless news articles have been published. Heavy metals also contribute to the severity of Lyme disease.

Because childhood vaccinations have traditionally contained thimerosal (a mercury preservative), it is believed that many autistic children were perhaps poisoned by their vaccinations. This is one of the leading theories as to the cause of autism. Although thimerosal has been removed from many vaccine products currently on the market, certain products still contain thimerosal, so you should thoroughly investigate the products you intend to have injected into your child.

There are literally dozens of resources available on this topic. The following books and internet discussion groups are among the most useful for conducting additional research:

Books:

1. ***The Top 10 Lyme Disease Treatments: Defeat Lyme disease with the Best of Conventional and Alternative Medicine***. By Bryan Rosner.
Paperback, 367 pages.
This book provides a detailed discussion of mercury poisoning as it occurs in many, if not most, Lyme disease sufferers. The discussion includes evaluation of various interventions, including DMPS, DMSA, alpha lipoic acid, cilantro, chlorella,

and more. There is also a discussion of testing procedures. You can find an excerpt from this book below, in this Appendix. Available from: www.defeatlyme.com.

2. ***Amalgam Illness: Diagnosis and Treatment***. By Andrew Hall Cutler, Ph.D.
Paperback, 226 pages.
This is one of the most significant and impactful books on heavy metal poisoning. A must read. Written by a chemical engineer who himself got mercury poisoning from his amalgam dental fillings, this practical guide provides information on a new mercury chelation method known as "frequent dose chelation." Many people poisoned by heavy metals have noted that this method has been the only one that leads to healing. Hundreds of autistic children have used Andrew Cutler's program with astounding results.
Available from: www.lymebook.com/mercury.

3. ***Hair Test Interpretation: Finding Hidden Toxicities***. By Andrew Hall Cutler, Ph.D.
Paperback, 298 pages.
Also by Andrew Hall Cutler, Ph.D., this book delves into the complex task of interpreting hair tests. Interpretation is complicated because heavy metal toxicity, especially mercury poisoning, interferes with mineral transport throughout the body. Ironically, If someone is mercury poisoned, hair test mercury is often low and other minerals may be elevated or take on unusual values. For example, mercury often causes retention of arsenic, antimony, tin, titanium, zirconium and aluminum. An inexperienced health care provider may wrongfully assume that one of these other minerals is the culprit, when in reality mercury is the true source of toxicity.
Available from: www.lymebook.com/hair.

Internet Discussion Groups:

4. **The "Frequent Dose Chelation" Yahoo! Group**. With over 1000 members and free membership, this group focuses its discussion on the mercury chelation principles discovered by Andrew Hall Cutler, Ph.D. Visit the group at: http://health.groups.yahoo.com/group/frequent-dose-chelation/

5. **The "Autism-Mercury" Yahoo! Group.** With over 7000 members and free membership, this is the primary online discussion group for communicating about heavy metal toxicity as it occurs in autism. Visit the group at: http://health.groups.yahoo.com/group/autism-mercury/

Tests and Treatment Options

Various methods are used to test the amount of heavy metals contained in the body. Similar to Lyme disease testing, these methods are quite controversial. Detoxification from heavy metal poisoning is no less controversial, unfortunately. The following excerpts from the book, *The Top 10 Lyme Disease Treatments*, shed light on the challenges of testing for and treating heavy metal toxicity, with specific focus on mercury poisoning:

Testing for mercury toxicity:

How do you know if you have mercury poisoning and how do you get rid of it? Such topics are subject of great controversy. Dozens of books have been written about testing for and treating mercury toxicity. Mercury "experts" vehemently shout all kinds of contradictory information at each other on a regular basis.

Testing for mercury toxicity is one of the most complicated and controversial aspects of dealing with mercury poisoning. Dozens of different testing methods are advocated. Most of the more common methods do not provide truly useful information about just how mercury-toxic someone is. Urine, stool, and blood tests do not give an accurate indication of the total body burden of mercury, because these methods measure only what are called "shallow" body pools of mercury.

One of the most reliable, painless and convenient methods is hair testing, because it measures a much longer mercury excretion period. But even hair testing is not completely accurate. Sometimes normal or low mercury levels in the hair may not indicate that a person is mercury free, but instead the converse: that the individual has been poisoned so severely that the body can no longer eliminate mercury through the hair. Interpreting hair tests properly is a skill most health care practitioners do not have. For these reasons, mercury toxicity should not be ruled out even if one or several tests show safe levels. For more information on interpreting hair tests, see Andrew Cutler's newest book, Hair Test Interpretation: Finding Hidden Toxicities, available from www.lymebook.com/hair.

Detoxifying mercury from the body

Mercury detoxification treatment is no less complicated or controversial than testing. Most techniques actually do more harm than good and result only in worsening of symptoms and minimal mercury excretion. Mercury is very difficult to eliminate from the body. Most substances and programs claiming to remove mercury, if they do anything at all, actually just stir it up and redistribute it to critical areas like the brain and liver where it can do serious damage. Using a mercury removal protocol that has a high propensity for redistribution is a very bad idea.

Eliminating mercury from the body is accomplished properly by a special type of chelation therapy. Chelation therapy is a method of binding heavy metals for removal from the bloodstream. Chelators are substances used during chelation that circulate throughout the body, bind to mercury, and are then eliminated along with the mercury they are attached to. In Greek, "chelate" means "claw"—the process of mercury removal is so named because chelators metaphorically claw out toxins from where they are bound in the body. There are many different schools of thought and ideologies about how to properly accomplish mercury chelation. Most methods are dangerous and incorrect. Below we will examine three main problems occurring in most common mercury chelation protocols and appropriate solutions for each.

1. *The first problem that can render chelators nonproductive and dangerous is that the chelator used does not bond strongly enough with mercury to remove it. Instead, the mercury is merely dislodged from its resting places in the body and sent into circulation, where it quickly bonds to tissues elsewhere. This is called mercury redistribution. It can have seriously damaging effects and can dramatically increase symptoms of toxicity. Body tissues themselves have a high affinity for mercury. If the chelating agent used creates only a weak bond, the mercury will be dropped by the chelator and grab onto other body tissues on the way out of the body. An ideal mercury protocol minimizes redistribution. Many of the "mercury detoxification" preparations sold in health food stores and by various healthcare practitioners are not safe or effective. In some cases, these substances and products can be very dangerous and often do more harm than good. Such substances and products typically create a strong enough bond to move mercury around in the body and cause mercury redistribution, but not a strong enough bond to actually usher mercury out of the body.*

DMSA (dimercaptosuccinic acid), DMPS (dimercaptopropane-1-sulfonic acid), and ALA (alpha lipoic acid) are three effective, appropriate mercury chelators that create a bond strong enough to successfully usher mercury out of the body and not just redistribute it. These substances have a long, established track record, and also have a great amount of supporting research. DMPS and DMSA are water soluble, while ALA is fat soluble. In a mercury removal program, both a water soluble and a fat soluble chelator should be used.

DMPS is a better choice than DMSA. DMPS or DMSA (DMPS is preferred) can be combined with ALA as part of a comprehensive mercury treatment plan. Oral DMPS capsules are much safer and more effective than the commonly administered IV/injected form of DMPS, reasons for which will be explained over the next several paragraphs. Oral chelators are always preferred over IV chelators. Oral DMPS capsules are fairly difficult to locate but can be purchased with a prescription in compounded form from numerous compounding pharmacies. DMPS dosing should be approximately 10mg-30mg, every eight hours, as described in the book Amalgam Illness: Diagnosis and Treatment written by Andrew Cutler, Ph.D. This book also provides instructions for combining DMPS or DMSA with ALA to build a comprehensive mercury treatment plan. More information about this book will be provided in a few pages. Some research indicates that building up from a very low dose may be the best approach to using these chelation agents.

2. *Another problem commonly encountered in an inept mercury removal program is that the chelator is not dosed with sufficient frequency to ensure that a consistent supply of it is available in the blood to "sop up" the mercury knocked loose by the last dose*

of chelator. Because even proper chelating agents (DMSA, DMPS, and ALA) do not create perfect bonds with mercury, they sometimes drop the mercury on its way out of the body. Thus it is essential to have a constant, fresh supply of chelator in the blood to pick up the dropped mercury and carry it the rest of the way out. Proper mercury chelating substances have a short half-life in the blood which necessitates frequent dosing (sometimes requiring middle-of-the-night doses) to maintain blood levels. One approach to safe chelation is to apply dosing several times per day. Less-than ideal dosing schedules include:

    a. Schedules in which a large dose of chelator is taken infrequently, such as a DMPS injection or IV once every week or month.

    b. Schedules in which a full dose of chelator is taken only daily or every other day.

    c. Schedules in which mercury chelators are taken on an irregular basis, such that there is no consistent dosing pattern.

3. Even if a proper chelating agent is used on an appropriately frequent schedule, a mistake often made is using too large a dose. It is not uncommon for mercury chelation protocols to use doses that are 10 times higher than they should be. The reason for using very low doses of chelator is that the eliminatory system of the body can handle only a small amount of mercury at a time. Mercury is highly toxic, and as you remove it you must ensure that the body has to deal with it in very small portions. If you take large doses of a chelator, lots of mercury gets mobilized, but only a small amount gets excreted. The rest gets redistributed and attaches to other tissue in the body, causing damage and increased symptoms. Larger doses do not get the mercury out faster; they simply make you more miserable during the process. A proper chelation protocol uses a small dose of chelating substance so that the amount of mercury knocked loose is easily handled by the

eliminatory system instead of being simply redistributed through-out the body.

To summarize, productive and beneficial chelation protocols use small doses of proper chelators taken frequently. Dangerous protocols use large doses of inappropriate chelators taken infrequently. Productive chelation campaigns result in mercury removal and symptom improvement. Improper, dangerous protocols result in mercury redistribution and damage to the body with very little mercury removal or symptom improvement.

These suggested principles of mercury chelation were discovered by Andrew Cutler, Ph.D. His book, Amalgam Illness: Diagnosis and Treatment, is the source from which to learn more about how to safely remove mercury from the body. Cutler's approach to mercury testing and removal relies on sound science and has been used successfully by dozens of Lyme disease sufferers. The book explains exactly how to remove mercury safely. I personally used Dr. Cutler's methods to successfully cure my own severe mercury poisoning after several other popular mercury programs failed to heal me. My hair test mercury levels were the highest my health care practitioner had ever seen.

The methods described in Amalgam Illness: Diagnosis and Treatment are not only effective in removing mercury from the body and reducing side effects during the process, but are also fairly affordable and can be used at home with minimal help from a physician. Anyone considering mercury detoxification should read Dr. Cutler's book before decisions are made. Even your trusted alternative medicine doctor, whom you see for all your needs, is probably wrong about mercury chelation. Mercury chelation is one of the riskiest and most complicated medical therapies you can undertake. Mistakes can cause serious suffering and sometimes permanent damage.

Although the methods described in Amalgam Illness: Diagnosis and Treatment (available from www.lymebook.com/mercury) will help remove mercury from the body, the process can take months or years. Anyone embarking on a mercury detoxification program needs to know what to do, and what it feels like, in the meantime.

NOTE: The above chelation procedures utilized by Andrew Cutler are not the "final word" on chelation. Many other useful chelation strategies exist. Please consult available literature and a licensed physician before making decisions on your chelation protocol.

Testing Laboratories

As we have mentioned, testing for mercury (and other heavy metal) toxicity is quite complicated. The two laboratories most often used, and believed to be most reliable, for hair testing for heavy metals are:

1. Doctor's Data, Inc., www.doctorsdata.com, (800) 323-2784.

2. Great Plains Laboratory, www.greatplainslaboratory.com, (913) 341-8949.

APPENDIX D
THE THINK TANK OVERVIEW

As we have noted, detailed treatment information is not included in this book because such information evolves much too rapidly to be printed on static pages. To access the most recent information, visit the LIA Foundation's website (www.liafoundation.org) and/or attend their annual conference(s). If you are unable to attend their conferences, you can purchase DVDs from past conferences at www.lymebook.com/autism.

This appendix will share a summary from a "think tank" held by LIA Foundation in 2007. This information should provide a good introduction to the Lyme-autism research taking place at the LIA Foundation.

Physician's Think Tank Overview
January, 27th and 28th, 2007
San Diego, CA

Written By Tami Duncan with
Contribution from Jeff Wulfman, MD

Introduction
The goal of this think tank was to discuss the link between Lyme disease / Borrelia and autism. Physicians were invited from all over the country to attend. The idea was to have a diverse group with many methodologies. The LIA Foundation wanted to discuss the best method for testing and treating this illness with the sensitive immune system of an autistic child. The following people were present and all contributed from their experiences:

- Tami Duncan - LIA Foundation President and Co-Founder
- Antoinette Grewal - LIA Foundation Executive Board Member

- John Kucera MD - DAN! Practitioner (Defeat Autism Now!) and Family Medicine
- Toby Watkinson D.C. - Complex Illnesses
- Professor Garth Nicolson -Institute of Molecular Medicine
- Anthony R. Torres MD - Utah State - Autism Research
- Nicola McFazdean N.D. - Naturopath and DAN! Practitioner
- Jeff Wulfman MD - DAN! Practitioner and LLMD (Lyme Literate Medical Doctor)
- Warren Levin MD - DAN! Practitioner and LLMD (Lyme Literate Medical Doctor)
- Kurt Woeller D.O. - DAN! Practitioner and General Medicine
- Robert Sands - San Diego Hyperbarics
- Teresa Yang, MD – LLMD
- Geoffrey Radoff MD (h) - DAN! Practitioner and Homeopathic Medicine
- Dr. Joyatsna Shah - IGeneX Labs
- Carline Banks - Patient Liason

Presentations

Tami Duncan - LIA Foundation
The day was started off with Tami Duncan, co-founder and president of LIA Foundation. The mission of the foundation was discussed, along with details on various programs planned. Each activity of the foundation falls under one of three categories; awareness, education or research. Tami also discussed the need for funding additional research programs.

Kathy Blanco – Mother of autistic children
The next presenter was Kathy Blanco. She discussed the present situation in the autism medical community, and the possible reasons for why most physicians do not consider chronic Borreliosis as an inciting factor in autism. It was emphasized that infections need to be explored in much more detail as the potential cause for autism. She also discussed certain genetic patterning (HLA-D4) that seems to be common in autism pa-

tients and Lyme disease patients. It was emphasized that there are many children who are very sick and need the medical community to open their eyes to this issue.

Anthony Torres, MD - Autism Research at Utah State (Immune Function Genes)

Dr. Torres discussed the details of the HLA-D4 Immune genes in children with autism spectrum disorder. He also discussed an upcoming Lyme project proposal. The project will consist of:

- Examining DNA from 85 families with an autistic proband for Borrelia b.
- Using existing DNA from 69 families (no autism in family) as a control group.
- Using statistical tools to analyze the data.

Funding is being sought from the LIA Foundation for this project, which is approved by the board but awaiting funds from fundraising events, grants and private contributions.

Dr. John Kucera, MD - DAN! Practitioner, Family Medicine & Holistic Medicine

Dr. Kucera gave a very detailed presentation regarding the present care being provided to children with Autism Spectrum Disorder. He shared the importance of "healing the gut" with special diets, anti-fungals, probiotics, supplements, fatty acids and herbals. He stated that it is extremely important to detoxify the child who has heavy metal issues with chelation therapy. Many of these children are harboring multiple infections and issues that need to be addressed. In regards to metal burden, he discussed the fact that mercury and lead, when combined, greatly increase the damage to the body. It was emphasized that in a child with ASD, the problem is more than just mercury. Other heavy metals, solvents, cleaning agents, fragrances, dyes, cosmetics, pesticides, petrochemicals, viruses, bacteria, molds, waste products, food additives, hormones, xenohormones, antibiotics and pharmaceuticals are considered to negatively impact the immune systems of ASD children.

Children with ASD present many GI problems, including diarrhea and/or constipation, abdominal discomfort, anorexia, poor appetite, lesions of ileum and colon, increased intestinal permeability, and inhibition of endopeptidase enzymes (dipeptidyl peptidase - IV) needed for the breakdown of casein and gluten.

He discussed a unique strategy for tracking success of treatments via communication with behavior therapists. Many applied behavior analysis therapists keep careful notes and tracking so that success of treatments can be noted based on progress in behavioral therapy.

Dr. Joyatsna Shah - IGeneX Labs
Dr. Shah discussed the details of each Lyme test that IGeneX lab offers. She explained the individual bands, their specificity and sensitivity rates. She gave her opinion on what the most accurate panel would be; how to interpret the Western Blot; which bands are Lyme-specific; and the quality control assurances that this lab offers.

Professor Garth Nicolson - Institute of Molecular Medicine
Professor Nicolson provided his research into Gulf War Syndrome and how Mycoplasma Fermentans is found at an extremely high rate in the children of parents with Gulf War Syndrome. He also presented research proving that a high percentage of children born to parents with Gulf War Syndrome indeed have autism (regardless of which parent has Gulf War Syndrome). What was most dramatic is his newest study showing that 58% of autistic kids have a Mycoplasma Fermentans infection. We discussed the different transmission methods of Mycoplasma Fermentans, including airborne, tick-bite transmission and more. In his research, he has also found Borrelia in

these children as well. His suggested protocol for treatment of Borrelia and Mycoplasma is printed in his literature available online at: www.immed.org. However, he mentioned the successful use of NT-Factor from Researched Nutritionals, as well as antibiotics. If a child cannot tolerate antibiotics, then herbal treatments from Rain-Tree herbals may also be considered.

Dr. Toby Watkinson- bio-electric homeopathy
Dr. Watkinson provided a very unique approach to treatment. Dr. Watkinson deals with difficult cases of many types of chronic illnesses and infections. He spoke about his techniques for unwinding the immune-challenged individual in order to bring about healing. His approach is not replicable by other practitioners at this time. Dr. Watkinson is working on this. We saw pre and post treatment lab work, which confirms that this process eliminates symptoms.

Bob Sands - San Diego Hyperbarics
Mr. Sands has worked with many patients with Lyme disease and Autism. He has extensive experience with both disorders. He discussed the exact biology of what hyperbaric oxygen therapy does and the most effective approaches to take with a child who has Autism but also Chronic Borreliosis (Lyme disease).

Jeff Wulfman, MD
Dr. Wulfman provided a very eye-opening discussion on the differences between Lyme disease and Borrelia/Borreliosis. The following is an excerpt from his presentation.

Lyme = a localized disease caused by a tick bite containing Borrelia. This can be eradicated by short-term antibiotics and may or may not recur, but short-term antibiotic use can diminish all symptoms. Tick-borne Lyme can progress to a Chronic Borreliosis/Borrelia-Related Complex state.

> *"Chronic Borrelia is an epidemic, which may be transmitted vertically or horizontally with usually no history of a tick-bite. This means that Borrelia is present in the body. A person with Chronic Borrelia may be sick or not. The condition of the host determines the amount of illness. In the immune-susceptible person, the Borrelia bacteria can be triggered by stressors - physical and/or psycho-emotional. Toxins such as metals, molds, pesticides, etc. can also trigger it. The other category in which the Borrelia can be triggered is by other infections such as babesia, ehrlichia, bartonella, mycoplasma, candida and viruses that cause a cumulative effect."*

Symptomatic Borreliosis is unique to each person and is multi-factorial with multiple-organisms. The condition of the host will determine how effective the immune system can deal with other infections. When a variable response to antibiotics is seen, treating co-factors may be considered to yield better results.

Testing discussion
In the think tank, the accuracy and flaws in testing for Borrelia were discussed. The following points were made.

- There are problems with current testing
- No Lyme test is 100% accurate
- The Western Blot is usually covered under most insurance plans.
- If a negative result is received from a commercial laboratory, you MUST re-test with a specialty Lyme lab that does all IgM bands.
- A diagnosis can only be made with lab work + clinical symptoms = diagnosis
- 20% of people with a negative Western Blot result are actually positive.
- Bands 18, 23/25, 31, 34, 37 39, 83 and 93 are specific for Lyme disease. If a + is reported on any of those bands, along with clinical symptoms, a positive diagnosis can be made.
- If a negative result is received, with strong clinical suspicion, then an antibiotic provocation test should be performed.

Treatment discussion
Several aspects of treatment were discussed, including antibiotic therapy, Chinese herbal medicine, herbal protocols, HBOT and the salt/c protocol. All of these treatments have shown some benefit in treating chronic Borreliosis.

With regard to the effectiveness of these treatments, experiences vary. It was mentioned that herbal protocols, Chinese or standard herbal, have brought about improvements; however, the most dramatic improvements have occurred when herbal treatments are combined with antibiotic treatments. With regard to the salt/vitamin C protocol, many people are showing improvements with this treatment. However, it is thought that the salt/c protocol is most successful in killing off parasites, which in-turn brings down the overall infection load of the patient, causing improvements. It is not known if the salt/c protocol actually works on the Borrelia bacteria or its co-infections.

The topic of severe candida issues among children on the autism spectrum was discussed. This was a big issue for parents who would be hesitant to start a treatment plan, including antibiotics, due to fear of exasperating the candida. It was suggested that a clinician begin a one-month treatment of Diflucan prior to starting antibiotics. Including probiotics would also be an essential component of treatment.

The ideal pressure for hyperbaric oxygen therapy was an important topic. With years of experience in treating children with ASD and Lyme patients, Bob Sands discussed a slow, ramp-up method for this therapy. His suggestion was to start at 1.2 ATA and gradually work up to 2.2 ATA. The number of sessions would depend on the child and his or her progress. He feels that a 90-minute session would be the maximum timeframe. Antibiotics should be used during HBOT to bring about the best results. HBOT should be considered an "adjunct" therapy and not a cure for Borrelia or autism.

Following are some general principles that may be important in terms of treatment:

- Clinical experience regarding how best to treat Borrelia in this population is early and limited.

- In this fragile population, it is critical to continue to emphasize that Borrelia and other infections are co-factors in the overall complex of ASD, not the only cause.

- An intact and highly functioning immune system is critical for handling the infections.

- Per the DAN approach, treatment of toxins, gut dysfunction, nutritional deficiencies, etc. are critical to a high functioning immune system.

- Based on studies of adult populations who have multiple issues (including heavy metal toxicity, nutritional deficiencies, and gut issues) patients may do better overall if these extraneous issues are dealt with prior to initiating anti-Lyme treatment.

- Regarding the order in which therapies should be used, addressing the current DAN factors first (digestion, nutrition, gut, yeast, toxicities, etc.) may be most beneficial. Then, once the overall immune system is in a healthier state, adding antimicrobial therapy may be appropriate.

- Co-infections must also be treated in conjunction with the Borrelia infection.

Goals for future studies

The LIA Foundation is in the process of raising money for an official study led by Dr. Anthony R. Torres of Utah State. The estimated cost is $40,000. Grants have been applied for and the foundation is holding an Improv comedy event with silent auction to fund this study. The study will determine the percentage of children with autism who are infected with Borrelia and/or other co-infections.

There are two other phases to the above study that will be conducted once the results of the first study are completed.

The group consensus was that an "informal" study should also be done among physicians. In coordination with IGeneX labs and the LIA Foundation, a minimum of 5 physicians will be running tests on at least 10 children and controls from their practices. Physicians from all around the country will be performing these tests to provide broad geographical representation. This is a preliminary study to get an idea of the percentage of children in the ASD population who are affected. This data will be presented to other physicians working with kids on the autism spectrum to encourage more research, treatments, and testing in this population.

Conclusion

In general, the "think tank" event was a success. The consensus among attendees was that Borrelia/Lyme needs to be considered as a potential cause or inciting factor in autism. More research needs to be done. More physicians and researchers need to be considering this and testing for Borrelia in their practices. Multiple infections need to be considered as well. Future yearly conferences will be planned for parents, patients and practitioners. These conferences will include a "physician's roundtable" in which more information can be shared with a larger group of physicians, who can then implement treatment strategies. For more information on the conferences, research, or to make a donation, please log on to: www.liafoundation.org.

APPENDIX E
MOTHERS' STORIES

The following are various stories from mothers (and fathers) who are caring for autistic children (or children with other developmental disorders). Please keep in mind that the authors of these stories are not medical professionals. Their stories are for informational and educational purposes only.

A Mother's Journey Toward a Medical Diagnosis for her Autistic Son

My son Alex is 7 years old and has autism. But what is the word "autism"? It is the diagnosis of a child who has deficits in many areas of social and academic skills, a child who cannot relate to his world.

But what if a child has these issues and also has other, significant medical problems? It is common belief that autism is only a mental disorder. In my journey with my son, I have learned that that is only PART of the answer. Autism can be a medical illness, as well.

Alex has suffered from multiple medical problems, from a very young age. With Alex, I had a child that screamed from morning until night. I was told it was colic. I had a child that could not go to the bathroom because of severe constipation. I was told it was normal. I had a child that had pain in his arms and who would cry and rub his hands due to neuropathy. I was told nothing was wrong with him.

I started to believe that maybe something was wrong with me. Why do I notice these medical issues with my child, while the medical community said there was nothing wrong? After all, they must be right. They have the degrees and experience. I am just a mother.

When Alex was 5, he began to change. His personality would go from being so happy to so angry for no apparent reason. He became extremely violent and had rages that reminded me of a scene from The Exorcist. Something was wrong. Even his teachers felt that Alex was in some type of pain, but could not express what it was.

I began my search for answers by taking Alex to many specialists who understood autism. They did all their testing and could find nothing wrong. Some suggested drugs to just calm him down. Alex began to decompensate even more over the next several months. I noticed more signs that something horrible was happening to him. At times, he had difficulty swallowing his food, and sudden, severe headaches. He constantly pinched himself all over his body, and hit his lower back and his head to the point where he was badly bruised. He would wake up in the morning and just begin to scream and become violent. All I could do was hold him and try to stop him from hurting himself.

I continued my search for answers, as I felt my son slipping away. I went to several hospitals, hoping for some type of help, but nobody understood. They did every blood test in the world, and said they could not explain Alex's symptoms. What was even worse for me as his mother is that nobody seemed to care. I would beg these doctors for help for my son. I pleaded with them to keep searching to find him help for his pain. Alex was a mystery to all who examined him. I went to gastroenterologist, pediatricians, two neurologists, a metabolic specialist and a genetic specialist. We did not find any evidence of anything wrong.

How could this be? My son was so sick, and there was more. He started to experience night sweats, trouble walking, and swelling around the face and neck. It was horrible for me to watch. My heart was breaking on a daily basis to see my child in pain. If he was normal and two years old and did not have autism, he may have been taken more seriously. Everyone seemed to want me to leave their office, or leave their hospital, and just accept that Alex might have to be put into an institution one day. This was something that I could NOT accept. My instincts as a mother told me not to give up on Alex. He was sick and we would just keep going until we had an answer for Alex's pain.

Finally that day came. I received an email from another mother whose child also had autism, but who was suffering from Lyme disease, as well. She suggested that Alex might also have Lyme, like so many other autistic kids. I wondered how a mother from across the United States could read my son's symptoms and suggest a diagnosis when all of these medical doctors that I took him to could not.

I sought the opinion of the last doctor that I knew I could trust, an autism specialist who was very compassionate. From the beginning, she said we needed to think outside the box with Alex. She agreed with the possibility of Lyme and wanted me to take Alex to a world-renowned specialist in pediatric Lyme immediately.

I said to myself here we go again. Another doctor will be telling me that I am crazy. Alex's symptoms do not make any sense. I was wrong. The new doctor was caring and listened to my story. He understood my pain as a mother. Alex trusted this doctor, even going up to him and putting the doctor's hands on his head, trying to communicate where his pain was. This doctor did not look only at Alex's autism. He saw Alex as a child telling a doctor that he is hurting and needed help. He diagnosed Alex with Lyme, and put him on a combination of antibiotics. His symptoms got 80% better from antibiotics. Finally, my son had relief.

Two compassionate doctors used excellent clinical judgment to figure out what was wrong with my child. Compassion and good clinical judgment should not be rare, but in my experience, they are!

Alex is doing much better today, and is still being treated for chronic Lyme. He has probably had this for a very long time. If I had only known about Lyme when he was younger, maybe Alex wouldn't have had these years of pain, suffering, and the experience that he was not understood.

If I had not figured out that Alex has Lyme disease, what would have happened to him? What about other kids who could be suffering, as well? And what about autistic adults, institutionalized for behavioral problems? Could undiagnosed Lyme be affecting them? I fear that because of the rise in autism, there are probably many more affected with Lyme and suffering in silence. Many parents and professionals just accept all behaviors and symptoms as part of autism. Even in autism, how can anybody think that a child screaming violently and beating himself up all day long is normal? He does not need to talk in order for me to know something is wrong. My hope and prayer is to get the message out to other families to check their kids for Lyme and to use the appropriate testing, to pursue a doctor who understands Lyme disease in its chronic, debilitating form, and how it can affect mental processes, including personality, as I had seen with Alex.

I know autism includes a medical disorder. Many of these kids are sick with multiple health issues. I now believe a chronic infection like Lyme could be a missing piece for some kids with autism. My son might not be able to speak, but his behaviors spoke for him. I am so glad I listened.

Thank you, Cheryl

Eugenio's Story

Our story is a rapidly developing one since our conclusive diagnosis of Lyme disease has presented itself quiet recently and I sincerely expect a lot to happen in the next six months as we plan to start new aggressive therapies. The main character starring in this story is my beautiful six-year-old boy Eugenio, our first and only child and a very enthusiastically awaited new arrival to my family.

Eugenio was born (in what, at the time, I considered a very privileged way), at the top-of-the-line Cedars Sinai Hospital in Beverly Hills. Only years later, would I come to understand that it would have been much better for him to be born in some small village in Tibet, instead of being welcomed in this world by vaccinations that his undeveloped immune system had to somehow make sense of. Yes, I naively thought that being delivered in the same place where Madonna's baby started her journey, was the safest and brightest starting point into this world, but I was wrong.

My little boy was born after a pretty average and uncomplicated natural labor and was introduced to me by the doctors as a very healthy, thriving newborn. Now, fast-forwarding in time to a year later, we see him growing beautiful in every sense and showing a very social disposition and great personality. We can continue going further in time and see how multiple vaccination shots have given him fevers and left me with a very uncomfortable feeling that, unfortunately, was not just some parental paranoia.

Eugenio at that time was reaching every milestone in time with the exception of language, which could have been something possibly explained by the fact that we are a multi-lingual family, with a father that speaks Italian, mum English and a nanny in Spanish. That was my theory at that time but now I suspect that maybe there was something more in him from the very start that had suddenly been precipitated by the explosive impact of the vaccinations . This something was not just some constitutional, underlying, genetic predisposition but maybe a dormant army of bacteria that was ready to take advantage of the right situation, using their opportunistic nature in order to proliferate in an ideal environment.

Now let's fast forward to a time when my wife and I are looking at each other in disbelief as we are given the life sentence that our son is autistic. They basically can't give us much help; as parents, we need to accept this lifelong condition and contact our regional center in order to get some support on schooling and occupational therapies. Eugenio was about three years old at that time and a strikingly beautiful little boy that seemed quite normal at a glance since he was happy most of the time, had normal eye contact and was very touchy and affectionate. It was true that after the vaccination his body structure seemed to have somehow switched from a compact, almost muscular one, to a long, excessively lean one, and his belly seemed to be a bit distended, resembling those sad pictures of starved babies from third world countries. But I thought it was just a transition of sorts. Of course we were aware that there was something very worrisome about his almost complete mutism, but we still were hearing stories about these children from bi-lingual families and their big delays in developing language.

But this era of denial was now over and we found ourselves with an official label of autism and a grim future for our only child. My spontaneous reaction to this rather overwhelming situation was to start getting information on autism and developmental delays on my own, since there were a lot of things that just didn't make sense to me. How was it possible that the neurologist that saw him last had nothing to say except that in her many years at Cedars, she had seen so many of these kinds of kids now, and she didn't know why, but it just seemed that a wild epidemic was going on. As soon as I started to research the subject I quickly realized that something was up since the numbers were speaking for themselves very clearly. In California, like in so many other states, one kid in less than two hundred has been diagnosed with autism compared to one in ten thousand in the days when I was born.

Ironically, just a couple of months after Eugenio's diagnosis, his little friend from around the block, who was the only one to come by and visit all the time, ended up getting his very own label of autism and was admitted to the L.A. schools special education program as well. Hence, I started to spend endless hours on the computer in search of some truth to all this nonsense, and the internet proved to be an immense goldmine of information. Reality started to become much clearer, and surprisingly, the people involved in bringing some light to this labyrinth of medical hypotheses proved to be mainly other parents who found a way to get actively involved in searching for the truth in what was becoming an increasingly controversial subject. After all, it was just logical that since our genes can't really change in twenty years, some other environmental factor had to be accountable for such a sharp change in the cases of autism.

Unfortunately, very few doctors and scientists seemed to be enlightened enough to study such factors without preconceptions, particularly when it came to reviewing something like the immunization programs they had been religiously protecting and enforcing. This daily process of scanning the internet, looking for all sorts of information took me everywhere from reviewing medical studies to parent forums and support groups, articles on homeopathy, sensory integration, and testimonials of recovery stories. Yes, apparently some people were lucky enough to have such prompt early intervention that enabled their children to resume normal development and step out from what is generally called the autistic spectrum.

Another truth that was also emerging was that every single child had a unique place in the map of the autistic spectrum and that understanding these peculiar differences was key to finding a way out from the maze. So I was trying to collect information in a broad realm of study in order to see patterns in the similarities and differences in all these very different stories, where so many elements were common and others didn't fit my son's condition. After a lot of time spent reading, consulting doctors and therapists, going to seminars and contacting parents who also did a lot of intense research, I finally came out from the fog. All autistic kids are different but all kids are intoxicated, infected with toxic metals and other environmental toxins. They all have dysregulated immune systems and suffer from serious chronic gastrointestinal disease. Following this common thread, you can find your way out of autism and move towards healing.

Once certain that autism was a biochemical disorder and not some inheritable psychiatric disorder, I started seeing a lot of different doctors; some conventional western practitioners and others that were following alternative paths like homeopathy and energetic medicine. This led me to meet with a rather unconventional doctor that took me by surprise. Just as I started to think of myself as one of those parents who have heard of all the therapies and theories available, I was shocked to find out that I wasn't. Dr. C was originally a cardiologist who, in order to find a cure to many misunderstood and hard-to-cure chronic diseases, had explored many alternative modalities of healing and developed his own protocol.

One of the tools he used to unveil what was affecting the health of his patients was a technique based in kinesiology called "muscle response testing" (MRT). With MRT, you can detect the presence of all sorts of offending toxins, viruses, and bacteria, by simply testing the reaction of the patient's system to vials containing a homeopathic solution of these. The practitioner, in this way, can test for allergies, toxicity and more by skillfully detecting a weakness in the muscle tone of the patient who is reacting to what is in the vial. Basically, it is a very quick way to know more about the person without having to rely on sophisticated lab testing. It also can detect which substances the body reacts to in a favorable way and can be used to choose the supplements that would be a good match for the patient's system.

Obviously, at the time, I was open-minded enough to go through such unconventional protocols and was confident in Dr. C's beliefs and skills; otherwise, I wouldn't have spent a day driving from Los Angeles to Arizona. Still, I was very surprised when his elaborate testing revealed not only the offending presence of heavy metals, pesticides and vaccines, but also a load of bacteria associated with Lyme disease. He specifically identified these pervasive microorganisms living in my son's body as Borrelia Burdgoferi, Erlichia and Bartonella.

How could my son have gotten Lyme disease? Wasn't that supposed to be a rare condition limited to people bitten by a tick in the woods of Connecticut? But with time, I realized that it could have happened many ways. For instance, my wife had recovered twice from what they called meningitis, just a couple of years before conceiving him and could have instead had Lyme and passed it through the placenta. Also, when he was born, we had been living in this romantic canyon within the city that had deer and coyotes.

I came back home with a very elaborate supplementation plan that would simultaneously support my son's body functions, induce toxin elimination and target the Lyme bugs, all at the same time. My son was also supposed to do a proprietary detox protocol called LED that involves using a tiny laser beam to bring the energy of homeopathically charged vials into the body to generate gentle but deep detoxification. Since I was already a

DAN (Defeat Autism Now) veteran, I wasn't intimidated by the huge amount of vitamins, herbal extracts and lotions, and I started to put the plan to work, eager to see some results.

Since my son was never a big responder to all sorts of supplements that we had used in the past, I wasn't expecting a quick, sudden reaction of any kind, but the opposite actually happened. My little boy, who is usually quite a happy and of enjoyable character, started to behave like someone who is possessed by a demon and needs some kind of exorcism! He would start running around erratically with pure terror on his face and would throw himself to the ground screaming, as he was taken by uncontrollable convulsions. His heart would race at unthinkable speed and he sweated profusely.

I had already heard about severe herxheimer reactions due to toxins being stirred up in the healing process, so I didn't want to stop the processes and instead continued the protocol. After a couple of weeks, my son's condition seemed to be escalating to the point where we were convinced that for the first time, he had seizures and at one point, he was falling apart so badly that we had to rush him to the emergency room. So I stopped Dr. C's protocol but I knew that what had happened was not at all negative and a failure. Such devastating reaction to a bunch of herbal extracts that were basically nothing more than some natural antibiotics, was proof of how heavily my son was loaded with these bacteria. The bugs were just fighting back and releasing potent venom as they were being threatened and dying.

It took months to rebalance my son to his former, more comfortable state of "unbalance." He was still behaving oddly and scaring us with his verbal and motor tics that would come and go, and displaying new symptoms and behaviors that thankfully, proved to be temporary. At this point I was convinced more than ever that Lyme disease was present and playing a very major role in Eugenio's autism and I started to research this field, as well.

Incredibly, I was to find myself entering another labyrinth as intricate and complex as the autistic one, since I was quick to realize that Lyme is also a poorly understood chronic disease and extremely controversial.

Here again, as in autism, patients are victims of a status quo which forces them to be proactive and undertake the work that is usually left to researchers and doctors. Basically, this was starting to feel like being in one of those "Die Hard" type action movies where the main character is trying to save is family's life and whenever it seems to be all over, something new comes into the picture.

I also was determined to have a conventional lab test with a positive result for the disease since it would have been helpful in convincing my more conventional DAN doctor and members of my family of the Lyme diagnosis. I studied the subject and came to understand that a big percentage of the people seriously ill with Lyme never have the classic bull eye rash described in the textbooks and also have negative lab test results. I decided to jump at an opportunity to get a tissue sample from my son's gums, since he had to have some dental work done under general anesthesia. I submitted this almost microscopic sample to a very reputable lab for testing. This sophisticated test detected the presence of DNA from Borrelia Burgdorferi and was conclusively positive.

Right after this, an even less specialized lab covered by my insurance, confirmed the same positive results for Lyme. For us it was a victory to know that a suspected enemy had now been unmasked, and we just had to hold on tight and pursue it until we would could find a way to defeat it. I never had accepted that I couldn't do anything about my son's condition and now it was clear that since he had bacteria that can have a major neurological impact upon their host, I could see tremendous potential to turn things around just by addressing it.

We are currently seeing some very good results by dealing with Lyme without having to employ the most commonly-used arsenal, which typically consists of heavy, long-term use of antibiotics. I carefully re-introduced the complex Dr. C protocol, this time without getting the same disastrous herxheimer reactions as before. It is possible that my son's little body is now stronger and his immune system more in-tune and capable of handling the challenge. I need to add that a lot of the things we have done consistently over the last years have certainly contributed to the improvement: NAET, Classic Homeopathy, B12 protocol and many others. We have more recently incorporated hyperbarics, colloidal silver and Amy Yasko's DNA designed bio- chemical interventions, with some very promising results.

Before considering using traditional antibiotics I am planning to do even more fine-tuning work with the natural options as well as do an assessment of the improvements we are getting. Either way, we are fully aware that Borrelia and the other co-infections may take years to be brought down and may never be completely eradicated.

What is fundamental to us is that we are now seeing a very consistent upswing in Eugenio's health and development. Now time doesn't feel as much to me as the unforgiving clicking of a time bomb but more like a measure of my son's continuing improvement.

A Long Journey

Who would have ever thought that time spent in the garden I loved so dearly would have caused us all so much pain...

I have always been a person who loves the outdoors. I have always spent as much time in my yard as I can. So, when I was pregnant with my third child, it was no different. During my first trimester, I spent a considerable amount of time working in my garden at our suburban home near Albany, NY. I don't remember a tick bite. I never had the "bulls-eye" rash. I just remember waking up one morning with extremely swollen glands in the right side of my neck, believing that I was going to come down with something. But, then it just went away.

A few weeks after that, I became increasingly fatigued and everything seemed to ache. I dismissed it as just pregnancy symptoms and never gave it a second thought. Then one morning, I woke up with what I thought was a pinched nerve in the right side of my back. I was about fourteen weeks pregnant at the time. I had a strange, tingling sensation which extended down my leg. I was told to lie down and rest, which I did. The tingling began to progress to all four extremities. The next day I began to lose fine motor function in my hands. I immediately went to the ER at a local hospital and was admitted to the neurology unit with suspected Guillian-Barre. During my time there, my symptoms progressed to include: numbness in all four extremities, face, and abdomen; tachycardia (fast heart rate), unsteady gait and balance difficulties; tinnitus (ringing in the ears); and a plethora of other bizarre symptoms. Around this time, my parents' (who were also my neighbors) dog was diagnosed with Lyme disease. I was convinced that I had Lyme disease, but none of the physicians felt that my symptoms were consistent with Lyme. Despite my strange symptoms, my tests all came back relatively normal. I did have one positive Lyme ELISA and one equivocal ELISA and a slightly abnormal white blood cell count, but my MRI, lumbar puncture, and nerve conduction studies were all normal. The Western Blot eventually came back negative.

The day before my discharge, I began to experience terrible head and neck pain and the left side of my body had begun to twitch and move involuntarily. I was still discharged and returned home. A day after my discharge, I was back in the ER. I had begun vomiting and was unable to eat or stand upright due to the pain in my head and neck. I had lost ten pounds in less than a week and the left side of my body was still twitching uncontrollably. They ran more labs at the ER which showed mild hypoglycemia, but were otherwise normal. I was told that there was nothing medically wrong with me and that I should "see someone to evaluate my level of stress". I was discharged from the ER and sent home. Less than 24 hours after that trip to the ER, I found myself sitting in the ER at a different hospital. My symptoms had continued to progress and I was becoming increasingly ill. My OB admitted me to the hospital for hyperemesis. I was given IV fluids and round the clock demerol and phenergan. I was given one dose of IV rocephin because of the possibility of Lyme, but that was not continued. I was stabilized and sent home after a few days.

Things seemed to settle down a bit after that. I was still tired and everything ached and my feet were numb, but the most severe symptoms had dissipated. I was still convinced that I had Lyme disease, but no one would listen to what I had to say. I had an old prescription for amoxicillin, so I began taking it. Within a few days, I began to feel better, but that was short-lived. After about a week on the amoxicillin, I began to have severe abdominal pain. Afraid that I was causing more harm than good and frightened for the well-being of my baby, I stopped the medication. The abdominal pain was gone, but my symptoms were back.

Not long after that, I saw an infectious disease doctor for possible Lyme disease. He ran a number of tests, including additional

Lyme tests. My Western Blot was "negative", but showed one reactive IgM band at the 23kd location. (I have since learned that this is considered to be equivocal by many Lyme literate doctors.) The lab also only listed the bands included in the CDC's diagnostic criteria, so I do not know if I had a response to any of the other bands. I did have an elevated ASO titer and was misdiagnosed with acute rheumatic fever and placed on low-dose prophylactic penicillin therapy. Life was quiet for a while.

In December of 2004, I delivered my third child; a beautiful and healthy baby boy. Other than being very jaundiced for the first two months of his life, he appeared to be perfectly normal. After his delivery, I went to see a rheumatologist because I was still experiencing significant joint pain. He ran more Lyme tests, which were, of course, negative. He also told me that there was no way that I had acute rheumatic fever. He informed me that I "had as much muscle tone as someone who had been bedridden" and that I should "lose weight, exercise, and come back to see him in a year." Needless to say, that was the last time I saw that doctor. Since I no longer had the diagnosis of acute rheumatic fever, I discontinued the penicillin.

That June I found out that I was pregnant again. That was the beginning of a terrible turn in my health. I began experiencing severe abdominal pain and diarrhea, tinnitus, major balance difficulties, spontaneous bleeding in my fingers, low B12 levels, headaches, increased joint pain and fatigue, attacks of severe hypoglycemia, syncope, hair loss, strange visual disturbances, joint deformity in my hands, severe "brain fog", forgetfulness and word finding difficulty, and many, many more strange symptoms. I couldn't remember what side of my car the gas tank was on, how to put the words together to say "chocolate milk", and even spaced out when I was driving and forgot where I was or where I was going. I was 27 years old at the time. I was evaluated for possible multiple sclerosis, lupus, and rheumatoid arthritis.

My tests all came back negative and my symptoms continued to progress. I spent a considerable part of my pregnancy on methylprednisolone (a steroid) and had monthly level two ultrasounds. I had to withdraw from my classes and quit working. I was barely able to take care of my children or myself. It was a terrible time in my life.

In January 2006, my daughter was born, beautiful and healthy. My symptoms never went away and I spent the next few months trying to continue with school at night, studying for the MCAT, and taking care of my children during the day, all the while fighting against my body and doctors who refused to listen.

By that summer, I had gotten to the point that I was convinced that I would end up on disability for the rest of my life, or perhaps even worse. I had seen just about every type of specialist that exists, to no avail. I finally saw a very kind immunology and allergy physician in Albany. After performing a number of tests, he concluded that I might have hidden Lyme disease and should go see a physician in Boston who specialized in the disease. I attempted to contact the doctor several times, but never received a call back. Desperate, I once again began self-medicating with some leftover amoxicillin that I had. The response was nothing short of miraculous. Within a few days, my mind began to clear. But, along with that, the pain in my body began to change. Instead of the intense aching, the pain became "cleaner and sharper" and the pain in my head and neck that I had experienced two years prior in the hospital returned. I was experiencing a Herxheimer reaction, which is a worsening of symptoms caused by the release of toxins by the dying bacteria. I eventually went to see my primary care physician who agreed with my self-diagnosis and began prescribing the medication for me. I was finally, after more than two years, diagnosed and being treated for Lyme disease.

Around this same time, my son began to display alarming developmental delays. He was started in Early Intervention when he was eighteen months old and began speech therapy and special education and later physical therapy. He had global developmental delays and hypotonia (low muscle tone). He developed reflux. He was irritable and would often scream out at night as if he were in pain, but no one could explain why. By the age of two, he could not even say "mama" and had begun to socially withdraw. His therapist would come to the house to work with him and he would lie on the floor and close his eyes. He refused to communicate with them in any way. I came across a study on Columbia's Lyme Research site and began to wonder. The study was looking at the prevalence of a Lyme-induced-autism-like syndrome. The children showed developmental delays consistent with autism symptoms, but when they were treated with antibiotics, they began to get better. Convinced that this was the root of my son's problems, I took him to see a pediatric infectious disease doctor at the local hospital. She informed me that not only did congenital Lyme not exist, but there was no way that I had Lyme disease. We left her office very quickly.

I began researching pediatric Lyme disease further and found Dr. Charles Ray Jones in New Haven, CT. I immediately scheduled an appointment with him. I took my son to see Dr. Jones and he started him on amoxicillin. The response was once again, miraculous.

My son went from being completely non-verbal, almost non-testable, and most likely heading towards an autism diagnosis, to virtually normal. We noticed a change almost immediately. It has only been about three months since he started his antibiotics and he now no longer qualifies for Early Intervention services. His language, which had showed profound delays, is now within normal limits. He smiles and laughs and hugs us. He is just a different child now.

Lyme Induced Autism (LIA) Foundation: www.liafoundation.org

So, this is our story, our truth. I know that there are others out there with similar stories. Until more research is conducted and the disease is better understood, there will be even more who suffer. These past few years have been a powerful learning experience for me. My hope now is to spread the word about the tragedy of Lyme disease. We are in the midst of an epidemic caused by a bacteria more sophisticated than our current technology and a disease that most doctors don't understand. I know that there are countless people out there suffering the way that we did, who are told that they are "crazy" or who simply have their symptoms dismissed as nonsense. I cannot be silent about our experience and can only hope that I can alert enough people to this disease so that they may not suffer the way that we did. Please, educate yourselves. Ask questions. Don't ever doubt yourself. Don't ever give up for fighting for what you believe. If I had given up or had not had the strength to fight and question everything, my children and I would have faced a very grim fate. I know that we would not be where we are today. So, please, don't ever give up fighting and help me to spread the word.

Peter

Our story started when Peter was about 4 yrs old, in March, 2004. After we moved from California to Colorado, we started having behavioral problems with Peter. Looking back, I'm sure it was the stress of the move that triggered it. After a few months, I heard the word "Asperger's Syndrome" for the first time. The more I read, the more I realized that Peter had many of the traits of Asperger's since birth. About the same time we discovered Asperger's, we also discovered the gluten/casein free diet, along with a dye free diet. Taking these foods out of Peter's diet was huge. I would say we saw an 80% improvement in 3 days. We also found Dr. Amy Yasko, and started her program designed for autistic children. We gave Peter supplements based on his genetics, and had a lot of success with flushing out metals and addressing gut issues.

In May of 2007, I was reading the post of someone who said her doctor had found 100% of his autistic patients to be positive for Lyme disease. I had never even considered that Peter could have Lyme. I was sure that he'd never had a tick bite. When I started reading about the symptoms of Lyme, I was sure that I had it myself, and that probably all of my children had it. I was right. We made an appointment with our chiropractor, who does muscle testing, and he confirmed that we all had the bacteria, Borrelia burgdorferi. I knew that the muscle testing was correct, but to prove it to family and friends, we had a blood test done on my middle child, and it was positive. With further muscle testing we also found babesia, bartonella, HHV-6, several strains of mycoplasma, toxoplasma gondii, mouse encephalomyelitis virus, penicillium hordei, rickettsia akari, borrelia novyi, moniezia expansa, coxsackie virus, and I'm sure there are many more.

Our chiropractor has a unique way of treating viruses, bacteria, and parasites. He uses a rife machine. He uses his rife machine along with a frequency generator and he can get rid of things, such as Lyme, in about 10 minutes. He can also test to see if the Lyme (or other pathogens) have gotten into the DNA. If so, he treats the infection again, this time for the DNA aspect of it. We saw some major detoxing after the DNA treatment, such as frothy urine (I'm talking a HUGE mound of bubbles), a urine sample half full of sediment, dark urine, etc....

My middle child has been sick since birth. He had a weak cry at birth, as well as colic, reflux, huge tonsils, slow growth, ear infection after ear infection, high fevers of 104 degrees about every 4-6 weeks that would last for 5 days. We had found some homeopathic drops for tonsils which helped a lot, but since his Lyme treatment he hasn't had more than a mild cold, and no fever (going on 5 months now). We recently took him to someone who has an Asyra machine for testing. It pulls the energy out of the body and prints on a computer screen all of the major issues in the body. We came up with many food sensitivities, african horse sickness virus, anthrax, borrelia venezuelensis, candidiasis, and dinoflagellates. I'm sure there are many more. We are just scratching the surface. We need to work on his gut and his immune system.

My youngest child has had no vaccines, and has not had any health issues. He does get a little congested when he eats wheat or dairy, but we are all avoiding those foods, so it is not an issue right now. He also had Lyme, along with all of the other infections, but his body seemed to be able to handle it much better without the vaccines that damage the immune system.

Back to my oldest child with Asperger's. Peter has made some extreme progress in the last 3 years. His biggest issue was always anger and aggressive behavior, but those are nearly non-existent now. He was kicked out of pre-school after 2 weeks. This was when we had first found out about Asperger's and we were just getting ready to start the diet and some behavioral therapy. After 3 months of behavioral therapy with an autism specialist, and being on his special diet and supplements, Peter went back to pre-school (a public school that had support for him), and they had no issues with him at all. He has been in a regular classroom ever since with an IEP, but with no real need for assistance. However, the behaviors at home have been a little more challenging. He would "let it all out" once he got home from school and we saw a lot of anger and aggressive behavior. We had learned from his genetics that the MAO mutation (MAO ++) was related to aggressive behavior, and Peter has the MAO++. Peter also has anxiety issues. And the COMT+- played a part in the mood swings. He also had the CBS++ mutation which means that his methylation cycle was not functioning, and that results in toxins not being able to be flushed from the body, along with immune system disfunction.

At the Lyme-autism conference in June, 2007, we discovered the Homeopathy Center of Houston. They mentioned in their presentation that anger issues can be related to the Hepatitis B vaccine, and that they have seen anger go away after this was cleared from the system. So, we signed up for that program!!!! Anything that addresses anger gets my attention. We haven't gotten to that clearing yet (another month or so), but I'm eagerly waiting. He was cleared of Hep B on the rife a couple of weeks ago, and the anger was way down until we let him cheat on his diet and gave him a few pieces of junior mints for Halloween. So, it looks like we still have a few things to address. The homeopathy program in general has been wonderful. They are also familiar with Dr. Yasko's program and use her research in parts of their own.

The other thing that we have done recently is the laser detox. This involved taking the energy signature from a toxin (such as mercury) or sensitivity (such as phenols) and shining a laser through the clear vial, sweeping the body several times, which causes the body to rapidly detox the substance you are treating. This is a method that requires professional supervision, as well as proper detox and drainage support. We saw big reactions to each laser treatment with Peter. During the first treatment, his whole body was itching. Other reactions to subsequent treatments included an entire day of nausea, a day of anger (from radon), and a couple other reactions that were definitely related to the treatment. Peter is one of those kids that never gets sick, so I knew these were reactions to the treatment. By the way, a kid who never gets sick is a kid whose immune system isn't working. Peter had a large build up of viruses, bacteria, etc. that his immune system wasn't addressing. Good foods and proper supplements will help.

The improvements that we've seen in Peter have been many!! He's had more frequent illnesses, and although mild, these mean that his immune system is getting better. Also, he has had decreases in anger, aggressive behaviors, and OCD behaviors, better focus, better social skills, and better overall communication skills. I can have a real conversation with him. He used to just get angry about everything. He does still have an occasional bad day, but that is a HUGE improvement over the constant raging that he used to display. I can now take him to places like Wal Mart and he is well behaved, until he gets bored and then whines to go home (normal kids stuff!!). He used to throw tantrums at those stores and once followed me around the whole store, kicking me. That's not something that would happen now. Now, when he does start to get angry, he is able to calm himself down. That is something he was NEVER able to do before. He used to only get more and more worked up. He was never able to self-calm. He used to be obsessed with Game Cube, and now he gets bored with it and only plays 2 days a week instead of all day, every day. He is still mean to his little brother, but it's mostly teasing. No more physical hitting or pushing.

The next, and probably last thing we will do is brain therapy. We have someone here in town who works with autistic and ADHD kids. She does exercises with them to retrain the brain so that parts of the brain that are not connecting can learn how to connect. I have heard great things about this, and I'm looking forward to completing Peter's recovery. I really feel as if we are almost at the end of our journey. I thank God for leading us in all of the right directions.

Robbie

My husband and I lived in the woods in Connecticut where I walked my dog daily or sometimes twice daily without any concern or worry that I would contract Lyme disease. When pregnant with my son, Robbie, I developed very low blood pressure and dizziness, which I attributed to pregnancy hormones. I also was so thirsty that I would drink two gallons of water a day. Then, I had some mercury fillings placed before I knew much about the effects of mercury. Within three months of Robbie's birth, I developed migrating joint pain and profuse night sweats, accompanied by extreme fatigue.

Within five months of his birth, I developed Hashimoto's thyroiditis and fine tremors in my hands. I also had air hunger and was losing weight, although I was eating a normal amount of food and was not dieting.

These symptoms got worse, and since I tested negative on a Quest test for Lyme, I was told by doctors that I must be depressed; that my pain was from holding my son too much, or that I was losing weight because I was not eating enough.

Later, I saw a doctor for my "depression," since I was scared that my own mind could be creating such terrifying physical symptoms. He told me that he was surprised that I was there; that I actually had symptoms that sounded like a textbook case of Lyme disease, not depression. He felt that the test results should have been disregarded, since they can be falsely negative and I had many of the clinical symptoms, minus a Bull's Eye Rash (which could have occurred under my hair or in any area that is not easily seen).

He was shocked that doctors couldn't correctly diagnose this in the Lyme capital of the world, Connecticut! Finally, when I developed Bell's Palsy, the first doctor put me on three weeks of antibiotics and I felt relief within one week. A week later I developed symptoms again and was placed on three more weeks of antibiotics.

I thought that my days of Lyme disease were over, until I had some amalgam fillings removed three years later, and the dentist informed me that I had swallowed some of the filling during the removal procedure. Within a couple of weeks, I became very irritable; my night sweats increased to the point that I soaked the sheets every night, and I was losing weight. In addition, I couldn't handle too much sensory stimulation and my focus was affected. Loud noises were absolutely unbearable.

After a couple of months of this, I went to a Lyme Doctor, had a very positive IGeneX Lyme test and began Lyme treatment with antibiotics. I remained on them for 9 months and during that time, started the salt/C protocol with great success, in addition to Artemisinin, HCL Betaine and Activator, Paracidin and Gallbladder Complex. I also take Candex and Armour Thyroid, in addition to Classical Homeopathy. Many of the symptoms I have had all my life, such as sensitivity to change, Plantar warts, and anxiety, are now gone. Given that both of my parents tested positive for Lyme disease and have had some mild symptoms like joint pain all their lives, and that my grandmother died of Alzheimer's, (which people with Lyme disease have a higher chance of developing), I believe it is truly a family disease. If it weren't for the re-infection I experienced in Connecticut, I wouldn't be experiencing the blessing of good health today. I look forward to the day when my children's children are born and will be free of the disease because of all of the work my children are doing to strengthen their immune system so that their children won't have to suffer like they have.

Now, on to my son. At birth, Robbie presented with extreme irritability, gastro-esophageal reflux, "infant acne" that ended up lasting for years, and irritability after eating, which I suspected was due to food sensitivities.

Robbie had difficulty learning how to suck, and had a very rigid neck posture that enabled him to hold his head upright at only 2 months of age. He continued to have food sensitivities that later presented with hives, but his allergy test came back normal. As a baby, he was thought to have a difficult temperament and a bad "temper", but I strongly felt that he was constantly in pain, mainly in the stomach area.

Although he wanted to be carried, his posture was rigid and he did not wrap his arms around us. At a little over a year of age, he didn't seem interested in toys until he learned how to spin them. He would make fleeting eye contact, but he seemed highly distractible and hyperactive. He had speech, but it was delayed for his age level. At 18 months of age, he started to become extremely upset at noises such as music, singing, and clapping. Any noise-making toy would throw him into a tantrum. The reflux, vomiting, and hives continued. We watched his diet and avoided wheat and milk, and that seemed to help a bit.

At age two, he went in for his "well baby check" and was 37 ½ inches tall, a whopping 95th percentile for height. He still continued to have reflux and hives at age 2 ½. In spite of this, he knew all of his letters and their sounds as well. He continued to be sensitive to noise and his sensitivity to change resulted in more tantrums than seemed appropriate. He also began walking on his toes. As he also had a new baby sister, we thought that possibly he was having trouble with the transition. We did note that he hadn't grown at all since his second birthday. He had had no change in his height for 18 months; not even 1/8 of an inch. By the time he was 3 ½ he had dropped to the 10th percentile in height. He also had diarrhea every day and fatty acid malabsorption evident in his stools, which was noted by his pediatric gastrointestinal specialist.

At age three, one month after a Hepatitis shot, obvious autistic symptoms began to occur. There was no mistaking it at this point. Prior to that, he had had some ADHD type symptoms, sensory issues and developmental delays. He started having massive temper tantrums, was hitting himself when upset, and repeatedly throwing himself against the wall. He became extremely hyperactive, had self-stimulatory behavior, was extremely phobic of door thresholds, people approaching him, dogs, and vacuum cleaners, and demonstrated echolalia- both delayed and immediate. He became fixated on parts of objects, wanting to sleep with paper clips, film canisters, sticks, and other things that didn't seem typical for his age. He was also very interested in lights and fans. His interaction with us was greatly diminished. He was having night sweats and hand tremors. He didn't seem to play with toys appropriately, wanting to stack them or line them up. He did want to be carried and held (it seemed that this was comforting for him). He would also grab our hands and lead us to toys, door handles, and anything else he wanted for us to do for him. He would flap his hands when over -stimulated and upset, and would also spin in circles. This all happened exactly a month after the shot. He continued to go downhill from there. His Lyme-infested immune system just couldn't handle the vaccination.

We immediately put him on the gluten and casein-free diet which resulted in improved eye contact, more appropriate speech that lacked echolalia (although it was still not on par with his peers) and interest in interacting with adults. He was almost to the point of where he was at age 2, with regard to skills and behavior. He still continued the toe-walking and reversal of pronouns, however. In spite of his improvements, in his pre-school class for special needs children his teacher said that he was the most impulsive kid in the whole class.

Three months into the gluten free/ casein free diet, he started to regress again. He started sleeping 17 hours a day and this continued, even at age four. He was in lots of pain and we ended up carrying him quite a bit. Then we put him on the Specific Carbohydrate Diet and he started to improve but still had autistic tendencies and OCD, with lots of sensory issues and hyperactivity, but he was clearly better. We started seeing a DAN doctor with good results. Still, he had massive mood swings, anxiety, and irritability and continued to need 17 hours of sleep a day.

I learned about the Lyme-autism connection and I listened for awhile but wasn't completely sold on this idea. With lots of encouragement from my family, who kept reminding me that I had Lyme disease when he was a tiny baby and I might have given it to him, we saw a Lyme-literate doctor and he was started on antibiotics at almost 4 ½ years of age. We also started a protocol consisting of pure salt and vitamin C, so that the Lyme bacteria would still be killed, regardless of what form they were in.

For the first two months on antibiotics and salt/C, Robbie had massive die-off symptoms with extreme stomach pain, frequent fevers, increased night sweats, incredible resistance to change, oppositional behavior, rashes in the arm pit and groin, bright red ears, increased fatigue and sleepiness. He lost his desire to do anything and just wanted to lie down and rest. But, thanks to the antibiotics and salt/C protocol as well as his diet, he started becoming more and more age-appropriate in his speech and started telling me that his neck, knees, and ankles hurt a lot.

After those two months, the die-off periods continued, but they were less intense and shorter. At this point, October 2006, Robbie had been on antibiotics for one year, and on salt/C for 9 months. It is so wonderful to be able to say that my son's Occupational Therapist is absolutely amazed at his progress! Prior to Lyme treatment, she thought he was the kind of kid that would have needed YEARS of therapy just to achieve only a tiny bit of progress. But, since treatment, he has made HUGE gains. He can sit still and concentrate and make eye contact now. Now he is extremely affectionate, and has even been discharged from

Occupational Therapy. He carries on complete conversations with not only us, but his peers, as well. He still has special needs, but it's more like he has some developmental delays, rather than autism. We are confident that the gross motor delays and learning challenges will be a thing of the past very soon. He is very empathetic and compassionate, and the sweetest little boy.

We are doing some homeopathy through a homeopath who works mainly with children on the autistic spectrum, as well as Neuromodulation Technique and Chiropractics. These things are enabling the salt/C protocol and antibiotics to work quicker and making everything come together. We have also started an anti-parasitic medication per our Lyme-literate doctor. The road has been hard, but it is really working. Our neighbors and friends cannot believe he is the same child, and my parents are so happy to have their grandson back. For us, thankfulness is an understatement!

Cassie's Story

Cassie was a sweet-natured baby at birth who seemed to be completely uninterested in eating. When I finally did feed her, she was incredibly irritable. I decided I would breastfeed her and eat only the foods she could tolerate. Those foods turned out to be only 6 in number and interestingly enough, did not include any foods with gluten or casein. She seemed to do well as long as I watched what I ate. Yet, she would have days where she didn't eat at all, had morning vomiting and seemed happier when upright. She also developed failure to thrive. I continued to breastfeed her with the limited diet until she was one year of age.

At 6 months of age, it was discovered that she had a golf-ball-sized brain tumor in her optic chiasm, hypothalamus and pituitary gland, in addition to hydrocephalus. She had two brain surgeries within three days; one was minor and one was major, a craniotomy that removed 60-70% of the tumor. As she began chemotherapy, she was not able to receive her vaccinations so her last vaccination was at age 4 months. She did seem to have some sensory issues, which she definitely did not have at birth, and she began obsessive behavior; repeatedly opening and closing doors, etc. She also developed auditory hyperacussis and mood swings. Her immune system suffered from the chemotherapy but we didn't suspect Lyme disease until the other symptoms became more apparent. She started needing intravenous immunoglobulin every three months and developed night sweats and fevers too, and then we started to think that maybe it was a mixture of chemotherapy and Lyme disease. Every time her Immunoglobulin levels would decrease, she would lose her balance and become more repetitive with her words and actions, and have pain.

So, we took her to a Lyme literate doctor and she is now on antibiotics and more recently, an anti-parasitic. She is also on the pure salt and Vitamin C protocol. She has been on antibiotics for six months and even though she needs another IVIG infusion, this time, her balance is not affected for once, so there is a clear connection. She is improving with her gross motor skills, as well. We are looking forward to her having a life without Lyme disease, something that is not only important in and of itself, but also because she already has to take many medications for health as a result of the damage from her tumor and the resultant surgery.

Mike

Mike was a sensitive child from the day he was born. He had a scary reaction to his first DPT shot at just 3 months of age. Not long after that, he was switched from breast milk to soy formula because he was not gaining weight. He developed extreme hyperactivity and stopped sleeping. Even at 4 months of age, Michael rocked back and forth in his crib all night long, batting a bright orange lady bug toy between his hands. By the time he was

6 months old, he had worn all of the spots off of the lady bug! Michael had jaundice that came and went, chronic diarrhea, and almost no hair. He went to the pediatrician's office for weight checks once a week. He had a "new viral rash" two, sometimes three times per week. Finally, at 8 months, he started turning blue while eating. He went through gazillion tests for failure to thrive, reflux, metabolic disorders, etc. and they could not find the source of his shaking/blueness. His behavior was deteriorating rapidly. There were days when he sat in the corner with his back to the world. Other times, Michael was wildly hyperactive, "high" but happy. We never knew from one day to the next, or one minute to the next, which Michael we would be dealing with.

When Michael was 16 months old, we finally found an allergist who nailed the culprit as some type of brain reaction to foods. Wheat, milk, additives, preservatives, sugar, many fruits, and corn were eliminated from Michael's diet. The results were amazing. Mike stopped shaking, calmed down, and even started pointing and gesturing.

His first two words had been "bus" and "truck." Now, he started saying "mama," "dada," and "sissy." On a low allergen, carefully restricted diet, Michael looked like he had found his way home. What we didn't realize is that we had been through the first siege in what would be along war to bring Michael back to us.

I have a video that, even today, brings tears to my eyes. It's of my daughter Lisa and her baby brother playing together on a pile of maple logs from a freshly cut tree. In the video Michael is happily following his big sister, pointing at buds and bugs, playing hide and seek. I wonder, to this day, if that was the day when he was bitten by a tick. Two days later, Michael had pneumonia. Just two weeks after that video, Michael had a follow up visit with his neurologist. He sat as still as a stone that day, totally unresponsive. Although she said nothing to me on that day about it, the neurologist had written the word microcephaly in Michael's chart. In other words, she believed that Michael would never develop normally. Then, following another bout of pneumonia my son was "gone." It took 3 years of ubernutrition, anti-fungals, and one-on-one to get him back. At that point, about 85% of Mike's autistic symptoms were gone. He went all the way through elementary and halfway through middle school with no label. He had periodic regressions which were always caused by infections or vitamin deficiencies, but which resolved pretty quickly. Nonetheless, there was always this feeling that we were running as fast as we could just to keep from going backward.

Then, one night when Michael was 13, he went to bed with a headache and literally woke up the next morning a different person. In spite of the fact that this personality change was accompanied by swollen glands, blue feet, pneumonia, and a plummeting platelet count, his Doctor wanted to admit him to the psychiatric hospital. I refused. I was afraid of what could happen to anyone in such weak physical condition in a place like that. Suddenly, I had Michael at age 3 back all over again. Sleeplessness, mood swings, phobias, facial tics, rigid thinking-all back. The pneumonia still did not clear with antibiotic treatment. Michael's feet and legs were turning blue. He had frequent nose bleeds, and passed out more than once during blood draws. Over a period of 6 months, we documented psychiatric improvement while on antibiotics, and rapid deterioration within days of being off of them. Finally, at age 13, Michael was diagnosed with ITP, IgG sub-class deficiency, and "some form of immune deficiency."

For the first time, a strong connection was being documented between Michael's behavior and his immune system.

6 months passed, with lots of additional tests that showed nothing. Michael's doctor got desperate enough to run tests for every germ she knew of that caused "psychotic" symptoms. Ironically, Lyme was not even considered in that list. Toxoplasmosis came

up elevated. Mike was put on botanicals to clear the infection. He got halfway through the treatment and had to stop because the herbs were irritating his liver. At that point, Michael had improved greatly, but he still had sleep problems, sensory issues, and a less than charming personality. I started him on True Hope vitamins at a dose far lower than what is used with people who have "true" bipolar. I also contacted a naturopath who prescribed BHT in a grapeseed oil base, titrated to Michael's body weight. This combination brought rapid improvement in sleep and evened out the moods a great deal. I added a cow based, enterically coated IgG supplement, and by now Michael gained some weight and had more energy. Based on Michael's remaining symptoms and a very elevated kynurenin level, (elevated kynurenin is neurotoxic and inflammatory. It's also highly indicative of Lyme) I decided to give Michael homeopathic Indole.

The key indicators for that remedy are being groggy in the morning, having a raised red rash on the cheeks, and constant motion of the fingers and feet. Michael had always had odd finger motions. He had been teased throughout middle school because he could not stop himself from doing these things, even in school. He also had facial tics which, again, he was teased mercilessly for. Within 2 days of starting the indole, the facial tics, red rash, and hand motions were gone. They never came back.

Mike stayed on those supplements for 2 years and was pretty much a normal kid.

Well, we wanted to try taking away the BHT because, long term, it's not good for the kidneys. Less than a year later, Mike broke out in a rash and started vomiting/diarrhea. This time he was hospitalized and diagnosed with Crohn's disease. After any number of treatments, all of which only made Michael even sicker and more frail (people with Lyme should not be put on high dose steroids) we moved from New York to North Carolina in search of medical enlightenment.

In spite of 3 negative Western blot tests, my gut hunch was still Lyme. Michael had improved on doxycycline, and worsened when he was off of it. He had tested positive for both toxoplasmosis and rocky mountain spotted fever, which made me suspect cross-reaction of inter-related species on the tests. He had taken-and flunked-Dr. Shoemaker's visual contrast test on 3 separate occasions over a period of 4 years. I had photographs of parasites on a dark field microscope test done in 1996! And Michael had stayed stable on diflucan for 3 years straight, with no elevation in his liver enzymes, and no deterioration of his condition. But I had been told by at least 5 doctors over a period of ten years that, "No, no, no, this was NOT Lyme!"

I finally hooked up with a DAN doctor at the last conference in Virginia last April. She reviewed Mike's tests and history, then tested him energetically for Lyme. It was her idea, not mine. I wanted to see what her hunch would be after she had reviewed the medical records, based on her training and instincts. So finally, Michael is being treated for Lyme disease and Crohn's. He did 40 HBOT treatments, which helped a lot, but the improvements did not stay once treatment was stopped. He is off steroids, off antibiotics, and off all prescription meds at the moment except Diflucan. He is taking teasel root and s. boullardi, vitamin C and sea salt, cat's claw, neem, and a plant based potassium supplement. He is getting VSL#3 and probiotics 11 from Nature's Sunshine. He is also taking venus fly trap. His weight has increased from 85 pounds to 95 pounds in 2 weeks. He has his appetite back. His GI symptoms are better and he is sleeping much better. The ulcerations that covered the whole lower part of his left leg are improving. His joints and muscles no longer hurt all of the time now. I would love to get the IGeneX test done, but I cannot afford it. I gave my house back to the bank last year and moved here with no job. I am working part time on the internet grading test papers. But it is worth it. My son is getting his life back, one inch at a time.

At this point, I see two possible futures for Michael. One is a future in which Michael realizes his dream to speak to as many people as he can, telling people that autism is a medical condition like diabetes, and cancer, that can be helped. Michael would like to speak in every state, telling people about what it's like to grow up with sound sensitivity, obsessive behavior, and tics, how he coped, and what helped him to overcome those issues. The other future is one in which Michael remains a chronically ill young man whose dreams are held hostage by Lyme disease.

An interview with a mother who played detective and found answers

(This mother also wrote a long essay on the Lyme-autism connection several years ago. The essay is available online for free at www.lymebook.com/lyme-autism-essay.)

Interview:

When did you first suspect the possible connection between Lyme disease and autism?

I first suspected this connection when I attended a lecture in 1999 at my local library, sponsored by a Lyme advocacy group, with Dr. Brian Fallon (who went on to become the head of the Lyme disease Research Center at Columbia-Presbyterian) and Dr. D who presented on neuroborreliosis along with its psychiatric manifestations and links to chronic fatigue, Gulf War Syndrome and ADD. Listening to these presentations, I thought about how similar my son's symptoms were to the descriptions and case studies presented. I realized that I had to explore the possibility of this diagnosis as a link to my son's difficulties.

When did you first "discover" the connection between Lyme disease and autism?

I discovered this connection in 2002, following the dramatic turn-around of my son that resulted from aggressive Lyme treatment using five months of IV antibiotics.

My son had been diagnosed with PDD-NOS when he was 3-1/2 years old. With intensive speech therapy, ABA treatment, extra-sensory occupational therapy, strict maintenance of a GFCF diet, and immune support from DAN! doctors, he was able to attend mainstream classes in our public elementary school with the support of a full-time aide. The aide was the critical link, as my son had behavioral and learning difficulties that would have required too much of a teacher's time to address. For example, if he were asked to participate in a group project in which he didn't care for one of the members, Kyle (my son) would simply turn his chair around. If he were handed back a test for which he had received lower than a B grade, he would throw it in the trash can. The less-structured classes of art, music and gym often required more hands-on aide support. On the learning side, Kyle's standardized test scores were scattered and indicated a wide variety of learning deficits, particularly with reading comprehension, visual-spatial, and auditory processing. The aide was able to address a variety of these difficulties without taking additional time away from the classroom teachers.

Following Kyle's Lyme diagnosis with a positive ELISA test, and beginning oral Ceftin treatment in the late summer prior to 4th grade, I began to notice many subtle positive changes. Kyle's 4th grade gym teacher remarked what a different child he had become over the summer. He now carried a happy, smiling demeanor, participated readily in all activities; and was much more physically coordinated. He asked me what psychotropic medication Kyle had begun over the summer. He was incredulous when I told him that Kyle was on an oral antibiotic. For the first time, Kyle's class photo showed Kyle in the middle of his group, looking squarely at the camera, smiling! Previously, Kyle had always been standing next to an aide, who had managed to keep Kyle (against his will) in the group photo, in which Kyle usually looked annoyed. More importantly, Kyle immediately began to successfully follow his behavior contract at school more than 85% of the time. Instead of breaks required every 15 minutes, which was his standard in 3rd grade, Kyle now only required about 4 breaks over the course of a school day. His breaks were usually less than 5 minutes and typically included a brisk walk down the hallway and/or a drink of water. His standardized test scores, and importantly, his reading scores, improved dramatically this year.

But it wasn't until the oral antibiotics were briefly halted early in 5th grade (because Kyle's father insisted that this was enough of the antibiotics), that Kyle became physically and emotionally very ill, and that we pursued far more aggressive Lyme treatment following Kyle's CDC-positive Western blot and erythropoeisis diagnoses. Kyle was treated for a combination of Lyme and babesiosis using IV Rocephen, IV Zithromax and anti-parasitic medicine at the end of 5th grade, at which time he had become too ill to attend school regularly and received outside home tutoring through the school. Kyle completed his IV antibiotic therapy in early August, a month after his father had moved out and filed for divorce. This family upheaval could easily have undone Kyle; however, Kyle went on to have the most successful year of his life during sixth grade.

Within a month of beginning at the middle school, all aide support was dropped. This took place in spite of the fact that Kyle now had seven different teachers and maintained a much more sophisticated daily schedule than in elementary school. He was fully mainstreamed and received all As and Bs on his report card, earning Honor Roll and Effort Roll status during the majority of his sixth grade year. He took all of his standardized tests with the regular class with no accommodations for the first time. He passed the Connecticut Mastery Test in all sections for the first time and his other standardized test scores showed consistent above-average marks. He played the clarinet in the school band and the wind ensemble. He became a black-diamond skier and a budding golfer. Kyle's entire personality and being had so substantially changed; he became a kind, cooperative, gentle and academically-engaged boy, greatly changed from the formerly impulsive, unhappy, uncoordinated, attention-deficit child that he was in elementary school. This was the link between Lyme and autism.

I realized that through the successful and aggressive treatment of Lyme disease that we had been able to improve the majority of Kyle's presenting difficulties which I had previously attributed to this label of "PDD-NOS". I have now come to understand that PDD, or autistic spectrum diagnosis, is nothing more than a label describing behaviors, whereas Lyme disease represents a potential etiology and treatable illness which can either cause or exacerbate an autistic spectrum label. In early 2003 (in the middle of Kyle's 6th grade year), I wrote a 20-page story entitled "What Does Lyme Disease Have to do with Autism?" chronicling Kyle's dramatic "recovery." (This essay is available online for free at www.lymebook.com/lyme-autism-essay).

I distributed this story to many of Kyle's former doctors – pediatricians, Lyme doctors, DAN! doctors – to inform them of this case study of a Lyme-autism connection that presented with far-reaching possibilities for others. Having seen what was possible for Kyle, I longed to be able to help other mothers with autistic spectrum children avoid the pain and suffering that my son and our family had experienced for too many years.

Why were you able to believe in and stick with the long-term Lyme disease treatment when it was viewed by mainstream medicine as "alternative", and when so many others would not have persisted?

In hindsight, the compelling reason for me to stick with the aggressive Lyme treatment for Kyle was that I, too, was diagnosed with Lyme disease in the fall of 2000 when I suddenly became acutely ill. Over the course of the next six years, I was on antibiotics more than I was off; I was diagnosed with the three additional tick-borne co-infections of babesiosis, Bartonella and mycoplasma fermentans. I consulted with two Lyme specialists and followed a holistic approach using aggressive immune support and heavy metals chelation before I finally became symptom-free and well. I was also a "typical" Lyme patient whose original diagnosis was delayed by the ignorance of my internist, a neurologist and an infectious disease specialist. I was able to rule out many possible diagnoses but these doctors could not explain my heart arrythmias, my severe joint pain, the tingling and numbness in my extremities, the headaches and "brain fog", the overwhelming fatigue and nausea. Finally, I took myself to a Lyme specialist and began treatment which gradually allowed me to improve. Because I personally experienced so many of the symptoms that Kyle experienced, and because I relapsed after dropping antibiotics when I had not been adequately treated, I could relate to Kyle's suffering and the need to continue long-term antibiotic treatment. The medical establishment's ignorance concerning the diagnosis and treatment of chronic Lyme disease continues to anger me.

One of the scariest parts of my illness occurred in 2006 when I relapsed with Lyme after a year of being well with no antibiotics. I am quite certain that my emotional distress over Kyle's condition and my toxic family situation caused my relapse. The best part is that I didn't deny the illness and symptoms returning (as I had in the past), but instead jumped on a blood test (which was

CDC positive) and immediately returned to a combination antibiotic protocol which had made me well the year prior. The scary part is that a month after returning to treatment, I followed up on a lump in my neck which I had been aware of for over a year; this lump turned out to be a thyroid nodule with abnormal cells. When I had the tumor surgically removed, it was diagnosed as cancerous and also PCR-tested positive for mycoplasma fermentans (even though I had been on an antibiotic and antimalarial combination for five weeks.) I know of too many other chronic Lyme patients who have been diagnosed with thyroid disease and/or cancers. Clinical reports and published research suggests a correlation between these diagnoses and that is what concerns me the most regarding Kyle's future.

Why are you now even more convinced of the Lyme-autism connection?

Unfortunately, we have not yet been able to keep Kyle well off of antibiotics, so each time we have taken a break, he has relapsed and progressed to former symptoms. What is fascinating is to watch the return of behaviors which I used to think of as "autistic". Now I have come to understand that these behaviors are nothing more than a coping mechanism for pain and unusual migrating sensations from Lyme. Because Kyle has experienced periods of "remission" and now knows his body well enough to understand what is "normal" and what is "well" (something that I believe he did not understand prior to sixth grade), he can verbally accurately describe why he chooses to engage in certain odd behaviors.

Let me provide a handful of examples. Kyle periodically "pumps" his arms with fists downward. When I asked Kyle why he does this, he explained that this was his way of coping with the pins and needles sensations and partial numbness in his arms. I find that Kyle periodically "picks" at his fingers during a relapse.

Again, he explained that this was a way to try to get back sensation in his fingers which were experiencing the pins and needles and partial numbness. Ah ha! So these are some "autistic" behaviors caused by Lyme-induced peripheral neuropathy!

Let me continue. As an infant and toddler, Kyle was known for talking to himself at great length in his crib during nap time (those baby monitors came in handy!) and other times when he was playing alone. I always wondered how this related to autism. Lately, Kyle has been talking to himself again. (He is currently not being treated for his Lyme infection.) In fact, this is now one of the "behaviors" that is being targeted for reduction by his school. When I asked Kyle why he does this, he explained that his head feels so swollen, that the only way for him to feel assured that the flow of his thoughts "won't stop" is to speak aloud. He is also concerned that he will forget his train of thought if he does not speak aloud. This explanation ties in so perfectly to the "brain fog", forgetfulness and word finding difficulty of many Lyme patients.

(An interesting aside to this word finding difficulty is that Kyle has recently reverted back to reversing pronouns, a problem which he experienced when he was 4 to 5 years old, and through constant correction and ABA treatment, had been able to eliminate. This is a common "autistic" issue; is it possible to re-induce "autism" if Lyme is under-treated?)

Sometimes I find myself reminding Kyle to stick his chest out and put his shoulders back and down. He tells me that he "slouches" because of chronic back and neck pain. Periodically, Kyle goes through periods in which he requires far too frequent bathroom breaks. For example, at the movies last month, Kyle went to the bathroom at the theatre when we first arrived, two times in the middle of the 90 minute movie and after it was over. Kyle was not drinking soda (or anything else) at the movies, either. At one point at school, rather than trying to understand that there could be a medical cause for this problem, the urinary frequency issue became a targeted behavior. Kyle would lose "points" if he went to the bathroom more frequently than once every two hours. Urinary frequency and urgency problems are common come-and-go problems among Lyme patients.

My last example...Kyle recently told me that he is having trouble with understanding his reading assignments and following the story line in a book. He reported that his eyes sometimes "jump back and forth" across a page and so his entire head must move with his dancing eyes to try to keep track of his place. I know that his reading comprehension has declined again. The decline must be pretty severe since even Kyle recognizes it. Since Kyle has been experiencing periods of severe eye pain and floaters for some time now, this reported reading dysfunction makes sense to me. Dr. Leo Shea, a neuro-psychological testing expert with vast experience in Lyme disease, reported at the recent ILADS conference that his testing will often pick up precisely this kind of visual tracking dysfunction. During testing, a student is required to read aloud; the tester often observes a student missing entire phrases within a line or skipping over entire lines due to visual tracking difficulties. This is a common problem caused by Lyme and its co-infections.

I hope that some mothers and educational professionals begin to see their children or students in a different light through these examples. It may be more effective (and will certainly improve the quality of life of the child) to target the medical cause of the pain which is exhibiting as "odd" behaviors, rather than using ABA or other behavioral therapy to eliminate such behaviors.

So how is Kyle doing now?

Unfortunately, Kyle is not doing as well as he should. Kyle is currently attending a small therapeutic boarding school where he is being treated as though he has somatoform disorder. This disorder is a psychiatric disorder, based on observation alone without any medical tests for support, and is diagnosed when the clinician feels that the patient has become too obsessed with his health and enjoys the extra attention that frequent somatic complaints bring. (This diagnosis sounds about as plausible as the Munchausen's-by-proxy diagnosis.) Fortunately, Kyle has physically recovered from his stroke-like condition which appeared when the IV antibiotics were abruptly halted. He is attending school regularly and participating in many outside activities. However, his academic status has greatly deteriorated and he suffers from many pains and dysfunction that disrupt the quality of his life.

How did Kyle arrive with a somatoform diagnosis? During Kyle's most recent relapse two years ago, the parents disagreed over the chronic Lyme diagnosis. The father pursued a custody battle to prevent further Lyme disease treatment. In the meantime, the 2006 IDSA Guidelines were pronounced which deny the existence of chronic Lyme disease. (CT Attorney General Richard Blumenthal launched a civil investigation into the formation of these guidelines as they may violate anti-trust regulations, and the IDSA recently settled with the AG and agreed to form a completely new committee to rewrite the guidelines.) When Kyle's IV antibiotic treatment was halted by his father, and Kyle was sent into a prestigious hospital's inpatient psychiatric unit for review, the hospital infectious disease "experts" denied that Kyle had active Lyme disease. The pediatric Lyme specialist who had been treating Kyle continued to diagnose Kyle with active Lyme disease based on clinical findings and that was supported by lab test results. But once in the hospital, the Lyme specialist's viewpoint was not considered. The hospital's medical experts could not arrive at any medical diagnosis to explain why Kyle suddenly looked like he had a stroke, talked out of the side of his mouth in a bare whisper, was overwhelmingly fatigued, was severely underweight and complained of terrible joint and nerve pain. With no medical explanation, the psychiatrists were open to creating a mental diagnosis – somatoform.

We have all watched as the insurance companies have tried to avoid paying for therapies and treatments under the "autism" diagnosis. For those diagnosed with Lyme disease, we have also watched the insurance companies try to avoid paying for treatments under this diagnosis. It is a shame that our legal system upholds these injustices and further upholds the ability of one parent to deny appropriate medical treatment to a child for a condition when differential diagnoses are offered. This constitutes medical negligence and abuse.

Prayer and faith have sustained Kyle's well-being until now. I am aware that Kyle is not the only victim of misdiagnosis and under-treatment. I am also aware of many who had been misdiagnosed for years who were still able to make dramatic quality of life improvements when the appropriate diagnosis and treatment was begun. I am confident that after a period of time, Kyle will be able to get properly diagnosed and treated for his condition.

I hope and pray that the long-sought-after "gold standard" diagnostic test which will undeniably show active disease will be discovered soon.

My Story in Summation

When my now 16 year old son was 14, I was frustrated. He had seen professionals his whole life: neurologists, psychologists, psychiatrists, etc. They were helping only a tiny bit. My son wanted to go to college and get a driver's license. He had diagnoses of Bipolar w/psychosis, OCD, ADHD, Anxiety, NOS, Depression, ODD, etc. He was in special needs schooling, and there was just no way he could ever live independently at that time. I decided to stop relying on all these professionals and do my own research via the Internet. What I learned was shocking. I first decided to have him evaluated for Asperger's. He was then diagnosed with such. When I asked his current psychologist how come he didn't mention it, he said it's not something he diagnoses. I was very angry that none of his professionals picked up on it. I had recently become a licensed professional counselor, and had thought about my son having Asperger's often. Counselors are supposed to let other professionals diagnose family members. I imagine this is to protect them, but this policy harmed my son. I also learned on the Internet that autism and related diagnoses are treatable and reversible, something also not mentioned in college.

I then started some new treatments on my son, and he also saw a DAN (Defeat Autism Now) doctor for some testing and recommendations. Within a few weeks, my son had dramatic improvement, and was able to come off of all psychotropic medication. Within a few months, he was able to do 1/2 regular schooling and 1/2 special needs schooling. The following year, he was in total regular school with no modifications and no problems arose. He is still totally dependent upon diets and supplements. I learned in my research that autism and many other diagnoses may be from Lyme. I had my son and myself tested, and we came up positive for Bartonella, and Babesia and low CD 57 white blood cells. Our testing has not come up positive for Lyme, but I imagine we all have it. Testing for Lyme has been a nightmare of begging doctors, changing doctors, paying cash out of pocket, and waiting for referrals, etc. I have learned that treatment for Lyme is such a nightmare to obtain, that one is forced to go to the Internet to learn what to do.

At about this time, my health was so bad that I could really barely walk and talk. I had too many symptoms to list, but know that I could not smell anything without vomiting, and was basically couch-ridden. I had a toddler and two twin infants at this time. The toddler at age 4, lost his speech, and the twins were behind in development. With biomed treatments, and herbs to kill lyme, everyone is now normal. We are still dependent upon supplements and diet, but I am hoping to one day kill all the germs and get rid of all the toxins and no longer be dependent upon supplements. What I have learned from the Internet is that Lyme damages the immune system, allowing other pathogens and toxins to stock-pile, and makes one unable to digest wheat and dairy. I have also learned that the health of mothers and children are very connected. Something has got to be done. I don't think the world can take another 10 years of the same accelerated pace of diseases that it just had in the last 10 years. Why isn't the government taking notice? This is an emergency!

Heidi N., M.S.

BioMed Publishing Group
2008-2009 Product Catalog

innovative resources for
patients and practitioners

The following pages are the
BioMed Publishing Group
Product Catalog. We hope you find
these books and DVD's to be valuable.

Toll Free (866) 476-7637 • www.LymeBook.com
For complete, detailed product information please visit our website.

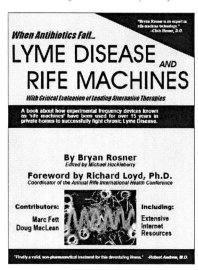

Book • $35

When Antibiotics Fail: Lyme Disease And Rife Machines, With Critical Evaluation Of Leading Alternative Therapies

By Bryan Rosner
Foreword by Richard Loyd, Ph.D.

There are enough books and websites about what Lyme Disease is and which ticks carry it. But there is very little useful information for people who actually have a case of Lyme Disease that is not responding to conventional antibiotic treatment. Lyme Disease sufferers need to know how to get better, not how to identify a tick.

This book describes how electromagnetic frequency devices known as rife machines have been used for over 15 years in private homes to successfully fight Lyme Disease. Also included are evaluations of more than 20 conventional and alternative Lyme Disease therapies, including:

- Homeopathy
- IV and oral antibiotics
- Mercury detox.
- Hyperthermia / saunas
- Ozone and oxygen
- Samento®
- Colloidal Silver
- Bacterial die-off detox.

- Colostrum
- Magnesium supplementation
- Hyperbaric oxygen chamber (HBOC)
- ICHT Italian treatment
- Non-pharmaceutical antibiotics
- Exercise, diet and candida protocols
- Cyst-targeting antibiotics
- The Marshall Protocol®

Many Lyme Disease sufferers have heard of rife machines, some have used them. But until now there has not been a concise and reliable source to explain how and why they work, and how and why other therapies fail. In the book you will learn that rife machine therapy offers numerous advantages over antibiotic therapy, including sustained effectiveness, affordability, convenience, autonomy from the medical establishment, and avoidance of candida complications.

The Foreword for the book is by Richard Loyd, Ph.D., coordinator of the annual Rife International Health Conference. The book takes a practical, down-to-earth approach which allows you to learn about:

> "This book provides life-saving insights for Lyme Disease patients."
>
> **- Richard Loyd, Ph.D.**

- Why rife machines work after other therapies fail, with analysis of antibiotics.
- Rife machine treatment schedules and sessions.
- The most effective rife machines: High Power Magnetic Pulser, EMEM Machine, Coil Machine, and AC Contact Machine.
- Explanation of the "herx reaction" and why it indicates progress.
- Evaluation of leading alternative therapies.
- Antibiotic categories and classifications, and which antibiotics are most efficacious.
- What it feels like to use rife machines – discover the steps to healing!

Paperback book, 8.5 x 11", 203 pages, $35

The Top 10 Lyme Disease Treatments: Defeat Lyme Disease With The Best Of Conventional And Alternative Medicine

By Bryan Rosner
Foreword by James Schaller, M.D.

This information-packed book identifies ten cutting-edge conventional and alternative Lyme Disease treatments and gives practical guidance on integrating them into a comprehensive treatment plan that maximizes therapeutic benefit while minimizing side effects.

This book was not written to replace Bryan Rosner's first book (*Lyme Disease and Rife Machines*). Instead, it was written to complement that book, offering Lyme sufferers many new foundational and supportive treatments to use during the recovery process. New treatments and information in this book include:

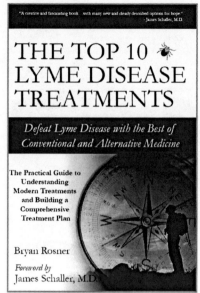

Book • $35

- Systemic enzyme therapy, which helps detoxify tissues and blood, reduce inflammation, stimulate the immune system, and kill Lyme Disease bacteria.
- Lithium orotate, a powerful yet all-natural mineral (belonging to the same mineral group as sodium and potassium) capable of profound neuroprotective activity.
- Thorough and extensive coverage of a complete Lyme Disease detoxification program, including discussion of both liver and skin detoxification pathways. Specific detoxification therapies such as liver cleanses, bowel cleanses, the Shoemaker Neurotoxin Elimination Protocol, sauna therapy, mineral baths, mineral supplementation, milk thistle, and many others. How to reduce and control herx reactions.
- Tips and clinical research from James Schaller, M.D.
- A detailed look at how to properly utilize antibiotics during a rife machine treatment campaign.
- Wide coverage of the Marshall Protocol, including an in-depth description of its mechanism of action in relation to Lyme Disease pathology. Also, the author's personal experience with the Marshall Protocol over 3 years.
- An explanation of and new information about the Salt / Vitamin C protocol.
- Hot-off-the-press information on mangosteen fruit (not to be confused with mango) and its many benefits, including antibacterial, anti-inflammatory, and anti-cancer properties.
- New guidelines for combining all the therapies discussed in both of Rosner's books into a complete treatment plan. Brief and articulate with step-by-step instructions for healing.
- Also includes updates on rife therapy, cutting-edge supplements, political challenges, an exclusive interview with Willy Burgdorfer, Ph.D. (discoverer of Lyme), and much more!

"Bryan Rosner thinks big and this new book offers big solutions."
- James Schaller, M.D.

"Another ground-breaking Lyme Disease book."
- Jeff Mittelman, moderator of the Lyme-and-rife group

"Brilliant and thorough."
- Nenah Sylver, Ph.D.

Do not miss this top Lyme Disease resource. Discover new healing tools today!

Paperback book, 7 x 10", 367 pages, $35

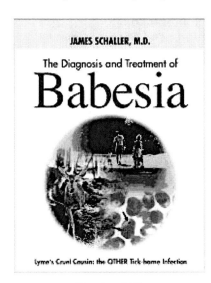

JAMES SCHALLER, M.D.

The Diagnosis and Treatment of

Babesia

Lyme's Cruel Cousin: the OTHER Tick-borne Infection

Book • $35

The Diagnosis and Treatment of Babesia: Lyme's Cruel Cousin – The Other Tick-Borne Infection

By James Schaller, M.D.

Do you or a loved one experience excess fatigue? Have you ever had unusually high fevers, chills, or sweats? You may have Babesia, a very common tick-borne infection. Babesia is often found with Lyme Disease and, like all tick-borne infections, is rarely diagnosed and reported accurately.

The deer tick which carries Lyme Disease and Babesia may be as small as a poppy seed and injects a painkiller, an antihistamine, and an anticoagulant to avoid detection. As a result, many people have Babesia and do not know it. Numerous forms of Babesia are carried by ticks - this book introduces patients and health care workers to the various species that infect humans and are not routinely tested for by sincere physicians.

Dr. Schaller, who practices medicine in Florida, first became interested in Babesia after one of his own children was infected with it. None of the elite pediatricians or child specialists could help. No one tested for Babesia or considered it a possible diagnosis. His child suffered from just two of these typical Babesia symptoms:

- Significant Fatigue
- Coughing
- Dizziness
- Trouble Thinking
- Fevers
- Memory Loss

- Chills
- Air Hunger
- Headache
- Sweats
- Unresponsiveness to Lyme Treatment

With 374 pages, this book is the most current and comprehensive book on Babesia in the English language. It reviews thousands of articles and presents the results of interviews with world experts on the subject. It offers you top information and broad treatment options, presented in a clear and simple manner. All treatments are explained thoroughly, including their possible side effects, drug interactions, various dosing strategies, pros/cons, and physician experiences.

"Once again Dr. Schaller has provided us with a much-needed and practical resource. This book gave me exactly what I was looking for."

- Thomas W., Patient

Finally, the book also addresses many other aspects of practical medical care often overlooked in this infection, such as treatment options for managing fatigue. Plainly stated, this book is a must-have for patients and health care providers who deal with Lyme Disease and its co-infections. Dr. Schaller's many years in clinical practice give the book a practical angle that many other similar books lack. Don't miss this user-friendly resource!

Paperback book, 7 x 10", 374 pages, $35

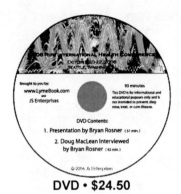

DVD • $24.50

Annual Rife International Health Conference DVD (93 Minutes)

Bryan Rosner's Presentation and Interview with Doug MacLean

The Official Rife Technology Seminar Seattle, WA, USA

If you were unable to attend the Rife International Health Conference, this DVD is your opportunity to watch two of the presentations that took place at the conference:

Presentation #1: Bryan Rosner's Sunday morning talk entitled *Lyme Disease: New Paradigms in Diagnosis and Treatment - the Myths, the Reality, and the Road Back to Health.* (51 minutes)

Presentation #2: Bryan Rosner's interview with Doug MacLean, in which Doug talked about his experiences with Lyme Disease, including the incredible journey he undertook to invent the first modern rife machine used to fight Lyme Disease. Although Doug's journey as a Lyme Disease pioneer took place 20 years ago, this was the first time Doug has ever accepted an invitation to appear in public. This is the only video available where you can see Doug talk about what it was like to be the first person ever to use rife technology as a treatment for Lyme Disease. Now you can see how it all began. Own this DVD and own a piece of history! (42 minutes)

Lymebook.com has secured a special licensing agreement with JS Enterprises, the Canadian producer of the Rife Conference videos, to bring this product to you at the special low price of $24.50. Total DVD viewing time: 1 hour, 33 minutes. We have DVDs in stock, shipped to you within 3 business days.

Price Comparison (should you get the DVD?)

Cost of attending the recent Rife Conference (2 people):
Hotel Room, 3 Nights = $400
Registration = $340
Food = $150
Airfare = $600
Total = $1,490

Cost of the DVD, which you can view as many times as you want, and show to family and friends:
DVD = $24.50

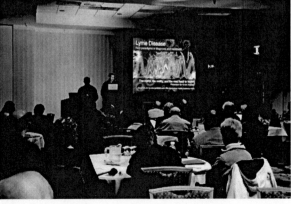

Bryan Rosner Presenting on Sunday Morning In Seattle

DVD
93 Minutes
$24.50

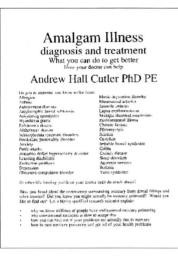

Amalgam Illness
diagnosis and treatment
What you can do to get better
How your doctor can help

Andrew Hall Cutler PhD PE

Do you or someone you know suffer from:

Allergies	Manic depressive disorder
Asthma	Rheumatoid arthritis
Autoimmune diseases	Juvenile arthritis
Amyotrophic lateral sclerosis	Lupus erythematosus
Ankylosing spondylitis	Multiple chemical sensitivities
Myasthenia gravis	Environmental illness
Parkinson's disease	Chronic fatigue
Alzheimer's disease	Fibromyalgia
Schizophrenia spectrum disorders	Sciatica
Borderline personality disorder	Gastritis
Anxiety	Irritable bowel syndrome
Panic attacks	Colitis
Attention deficit hyperactivity disorder	Crohn's disease
Learning disabilities	Sleep disorders
Endocrine problems	Anorexia nervosa
Depression	Bulimia
Obsessive-compulsive disorder	Tics	Tourette syndrome

Or other life limiting problem your doctor can't do much about?

Have you heard about the controversy surrounding mercury from dental fillings and other sources? Did you know you might actually be mercury poisoned? Would you like so find out? Let a highly qualified research scientist explain:

- why we know millions of people have and against mercury poisoning
- why conventional medicine is slow to accept this
- how you can find out if your problems are actually due to mercury
- how to cure mercury poisoning and get rid of your health problems

Book • $35

Amalgam Illness, Diagnosis and Treatment: What You Can Do to Get Better, How Your Doctor Can Help

By Andrew Cutler, PhD

This book was written by a chemical engineer who himself got mercury poisoning from his amalgam dental fillings. He found that there was no suitable educational material for either the patient or the physician. Knowing how much people can suffer from this condition, he wrote this book to help them get well. With a PhD in chemistry from Princeton University and extensive study in biochemistry and medicine, Andrew Cutler uses layman's terms to explain how people become mercury poisoned and what to do about it. Mercury poisoning can easily be cured with over-the-counter oral chelators – this book explains how.

In the book you will find practical guidance on how to tell if you really have chronic mercury poisoning or some other problem. Proper diagnostic procedures are provided so that sick people can decide what is wrong rather than trying random treatments. If mercury poisoning is your problem, the book tells you how to get the mercury out of your body, and how to feel good while you do that. The treatment section gives step-by-step directions to figure out exactly what mercury is doing to you and how to fix it.

"Dr. Cutler uses his background in chemistry to explain the safest approach to treat mercury poisoning. I am a physician and am personally using his protocol on myself."

- Melissa Myers, M.D.

Sections also explain how the scientific literature shows many people must be getting poisoned by their amalgam fillings, why such a regulatory blunder occurred, and how the debate between "mainstream" and "alternative" medicine makes it more difficult for you to get the medical help you need.

This down-to-earth book lets patients take care of themselves. It also lets doctors who are not familiar with chronic mercury intoxication treat it. The book is a practical guide to getting well. Sample sections from the book:

- Why worry about mercury poisoning?
- What mercury does to you – symptoms, laboratory test irregularities, diagnostic checklist.
- How to treat mercury poisoning easily with oral chelators.
- Dealing with other metals including copper, arsenic, lead, cadmium.
- Dietary and supplement guidelines.
- Balancing hormones during the recovery process.
- How to feel good while you are chelating the metals out.
- How heavy metals cause infections to thrive in the body.
- Politics and mercury.

This is the world's most authoritative, accurate book on mercury poisoning.

Paperback book, 8.5 x 11", 226 pages, $35

Hair Test Interpretation: Finding Hidden Toxicities

By Andrew Cutler, PhD

Hair tests are worth doing because a surprising number of people diagnosed with incurable chronic health conditions actually turn out to have a heavy metal problem; quite often, mercury poisoning. Heavy metal problems are easy to correct. Hair testing allows the underlying problem to be identified – and the chronic health condition often disappears with proper detoxification.

Hair Test Interpretation: Finding Hidden Toxicities is a practical book that explains how to interpret **Doctor's Data, Inc**. and **Great Plains Laboratory** hair tests. A step-by-step discussion is provided, with figures to illustrate the process and make it easy. The book gives examples using actual hair test results from real people.

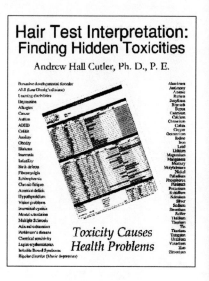

Hair Test Interpretation: Finding Hidden Toxicities

Andrew Hall Cutler, Ph. D., P. E.

Toxicity Causes Health Problems

Book • $35

One of the problems with hair testing is that both conventional and alternative health care providers do not know how to interpret these tests. Interpretation is not as simple as looking at the results and assuming that any mineral out of the reference range is a problem mineral.

Interpretation is complicated because heavy metal toxicity, especially mercury poisoning, interferes with mineral transport throughout the body. Ironically, if someone is mercury poisoned, hair test mercury is often low and other minerals may be elevated or take on unusual values. For example, mercury often causes retention of

"This new book of Andrew's is the definitive guide in the confusing world of heavy metal poisoning diagnosis and treatment. I'm a practicing physician, 20 years now, specializing in detoxification programs for treatment of resistant conditions. It was fairly difficult to diagnose these heavy metal conditions before I met Andrew Cutler and developed a close relationship with him while reading his books. In this book I found his usual painful attention to detail gave a solid framework for understanding the complexity of mercury toxicity as well as the less common exposures. You really couldn't ask for a better reference book on a subject most researchers and physicians are still fumbling in the dark about."
- **Dr. Rick Marschall**

arsenic, antimony, tin, titanium, zirconium, and aluminum. An inexperienced health care provider may wrongfully assume that one of these other minerals is the culprit, when in reality mercury is the true toxicity.

So, as you can see, getting a hair test is only the first step. The second step is figuring out what the hair test means. Andrew Cutler, PhD, is a registered professional chemical engineer with years of experience in biochemical and healthcare research. This clear and concise book makes hair test interpretation easy, so that you know which toxicities are causing your health problems.

Paperback book, 8.5 x 11", 298 pages, $35

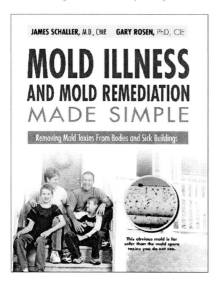

JAMES SCHALLER, M.D., CMR   GARY ROSEN, PhD, CIE

MOLD ILLNESS
AND MOLD REMEDIATION
MADE SIMPLE

Removing Mold Toxins From Bodies and Sick Buildings

This obvious mold is far safer than the mold spore toxins you do not see.

Book • $26.50

Mold Illness and Mold Remediation Made Simple: Removing Mold Toxins from Bodies and Sick Buildings

By James Schaller, M.D. and Gary Rosen, Ph.D.

Indoor mold toxins are much more dangerous and prevalent than most people realize. Visible mold in and around your house is far less dangerous than the mold you cannot see. Indoor mold toxicity, in addition to causing its own unique set of health problems and symptoms, also greatly contributes to the severity of most chronic illnesses.

In this book, a top physician and experienced contractor team up to help you quickly recover from indoor mold exposure. This book is easy to read with many color photographs and illustrations.

Dr. Schaller is a practicing physician in Florida who has written more than 15 books. He is one of the few physicians in the United States successfully treating mold toxin illness in children and adults.

Dr. Rosen is a biochemist with training under a Nobel Prize winning researcher at UCLA. He has written several books and is an expert in the mold remediation of homes. Dr. Rosen and his family are sensitive to mold toxins so he writes not only from professional experience, but also from personal experience.

Together, the two authors have certification in mold testing, mold remediation, and indoor environmental health. This book is one of the most complete on the subject, and includes discussion of the following topics:

- Potential mold problems encountered in new homes, schools, and jobs.
- Diagnosing mold illness.
- Mold as it relates to dryness and humidity.
- Mold toxins and cancer treatment.
- Mold toxins and relationships.
- Crawlspaces, basements, attics, home cleaning techniques, and vacuums.
- Training your eyes to discern indoor mold.
- Leptin and obesity.
- Appropriate/inappropriate air filters and cleaners.
- How to handle old, musty products, materials and books, and how to safely sterilize them.
- A description of various types of molds, images of them, and their relative toxicity.
- Blood testing and how to use it to find hidden health problems.
- The book is written in a friendly, casual tone that allows easy comprehension and information retention.

> "A concise, practical guide on dealing with mold toxins and their effects."
>
> **- Bryan Rosner**

Many people are affected by mold toxins. Are you? If you can find a smarter or clearer book on this subject, buy it!

Paperback book, 8.5 x 11", 140 pages, $26.50

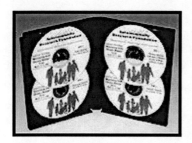

4-DVD Set • $45

Marshall Protocol 4-DVD Set

Recent Chicago Conference:
"Recovering from Chronic Disease"
Recent Hartford Conference:
"30th Anniversary of Lyme"

The Marshall Protocol is not just important, but critical in Lyme Disease recovery. It addresses a part of the Lyme Disease complex that no other treatment, protocol, diet, or supplement can even come close to touching: infection with cell-wall-deficient bacteria.

Borrelia Burgdorferi, the causative bacteria in Lyme Disease, comes in three forms: spirochete, cyst, and cell-wall-deficient. All forms must be addressed to achieve a complete recovery. Spirochetes are successfully killed by rife technology. Cysts can be killed by certain antibiotics (including 5-nitromidizoles and hydroxychloroquine). Cysts can also be exposed and killed by rife therapy with proper treatment timing and planning. However, until the Marshall Protocol, there was not an effective treatment for cell-wall-deficient bacteria.

Conventionally, doctors have tried to use certain types of antibiotics to kill cell-wall-deficient bacteria. Top choices include protein synthesis inhibitors such as the macrolides (Zithromax and Biaxin), the ketolides (Ketek), and the tetracyclines (tetracycline, doxycycline, and minocycline). Unfortunately, these antibiotics have been ineffective at worst and only moderately effective at best. According to new research and user reports, the Marshall Protocol successfully targets and kills these cell-wall-deficient bacteria.

> "The Marshall Protocol – especially when combined with rife therapy – fills an important gap in existing Lyme treatment."
> - Bryan Rosner

This 4-DVD set is exclusively offered by lymebook.com. It was assembled for lymebook.com by the founder of the Autoimmunity Research Foundation, Trevor Marshall, PhD, who also invented the protocol. The DVD set includes video recordings from two conferences of particular interest to Lyme sufferers:

- **DVD 1**: 30th Anniversary of Lyme – Hartford, Connecticut
- **DVD 2-4**: Recovering from Chronic Disease – Chicago, Illinois

James P   Leonard   Lida H   Janet
Kiley, PhD   Jason, PhD   Mattman, PhD   Whitley, PhD

Conference Speakers

Andrew   Trevor G   Meg
Wright, MD   Marshall, PhD   Mangin, RN

4-DVD Set

12+ hours of viewing

Coverage of two Conferences

$45

Researching the Marshall Protocol is an Essential Part of Your Lyme Disease Education!

Physicians Desk Reference (PDR) Books

Most people have heard of *Physicians Desk Reference* (PDR) because, for over 60 years, physicians and researchers have turned to PDR for the latest word on prescription drugs. Today, PDR is considered the standard prescription drug reference and can be found in virtually every physician's office, hospital, and pharmacy in the United States. In fact, nine out of 10 doctors consider PDR their most important drug information reference source. The current edition is over 3,500 pages long (with a full color directory) and weighs more than 5 lbs. It includes comprehensive and up-to-date information on more than 4,000 FDA-approved drugs.

You may not know that Thomson Healthcare, publisher of PDR, offers PDR reference books not only for drugs, but also for herbal and nutritional supplements. No other available books come even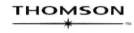
close to the amount of information provided in these PDRs—*PDR for Herbal Medicines* weighs 5 lbs and has over 900 pages, and *PDR for Nutritional Supplements* weighs over 3 lbs and has more than 500 pages.

Lymebook.com carries all three PDRs: *PDR for Prescription Drugs, PDR for Herbal Medicines,* and *PDR for Nutritional Supplements.* Although PDR books are typically used by healthcare practitioners, we feel that these resources are also essential for people interested in or recovering from chronic disease. Ownership of PDR books allows you to have at your fingertips information that has historically not been available to the public. Health decisions are always made based on information, and we want you to have the most complete information available.

Would you like to be able to look up all the details of the treatments you are using (or planning to use)? PDR reference books offer the following data on thousands of herbs, supplements and drugs:

- Description and method of action
- Pharmacology
- Available trade names / brands
- Indications and usage
- Research summaries, with recent scientific studies and clinical results
- Contraindications, precautions, adverse reactions

- How supplied
- Scientific literature overviews
- Dosage and administration
- History of use
- Biochemistry and metabolism
- Pharmacokinetics
- Cross references to other helpful data relating to the drug or herb discussed

The PDRs organize the supplements, herbs, and medicines in numerous ways, so you can quickly and easily find the information you need. Multiple color-coded, photo-supported indexes are provided. Supplements and drugs are categorized according to type, name, and health condition, among other differentiators.

> "I relied heavily on the PDRs during the research phase of writing my books. Without these books, I'm not sure I could have pulled together the information I needed."
>
> - Bryan Rosner

In addition to information about individual herbs, supplements, and drugs, the PDRs also provide high-level comprehensive health resources such as breakthroughs in the treatment of specific health conditions, anti-aging science, cancer studies, sports medicine, nutrition, and much more.

If you are a doctor, nurse, holistic healthcare provider, or simply a patient wishing to do your own research, these books are must-have resources. They pay for themselves many times over after years of use as reliable reference guides.

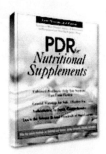

PDR for Nutritional Supplements

This PDR focuses on the following types of supplements:

- Vitamins
- Minerals
- Amino acids
- Hormones
- Lipids
- Glyconutrients
- Probiotics
- Proteins
- Many more!

"In a part of the health field not known for its devotion to rigorous science, [this book] brings to the practitioner and the curious patient a wealth of hard facts."

- Roger Guillemin, M.D., Ph.D., Nobel Laureate in Physiology and Medicine

Book • $69.50

The book also suggests supplements that can help reduce prescription drug side effects, has full-color photographs of various popular commercial formulations (and contact information for the associated suppliers), and so much more! Become educated instead of guessing which supplements to take.

Hardcover book, 11 x 9.3", 575 pages, $69.50

PDR for Herbal Medicines

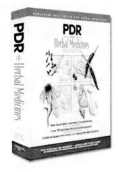

PDR for Herbal Medicines is very well organized and presents information on hundreds of common and uncommon herbs and herbal preparations. Indications and usage are examined with regard to homeopathy, Indian and Chinese medicine, and unproven (yet popular) applications.

In an area of healthcare so unstudied and vulnerable to hearsay and hype, this scientifically referenced book allows you to find out the real story behind the herbs lining the walls of your local health food store.

Use this reference before spending money on herbal products!

Book • $69.50

Hardcover book, 11 x 9.3", 988 pages, $69.50

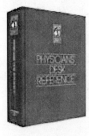

PDR for Prescription Drugs

With more than 3,000 pages, this is the most comprehensive and respected book in the world on over 4,000 drugs. Drugs are indexed by both brand and generic name (in the same convenient index) and also by manufacturer and product category. This PDR provides usage information and warnings, drug interactions, plus a detailed, full-color directory with descriptions and cross references for the drugs. A new format allows dramatically improved readability and easier access to the information you need now.

Book • $99.50

Hardcover book, 12.5 x 9.5", 3533 pages, $99.50

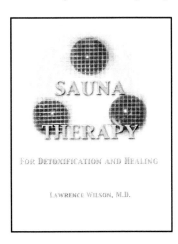

Book • $19.95

Sauna Therapy for Detoxification and Healing

By Lawrence Wilson, MD

This book is the single most authoritative source on sauna therapy. It includes construction plans for a low-cost electric light sauna. The book is well referenced with an extensive bibliography.

Sauna therapy, especially with an electric light sauna, is one of the most powerful, safe and cost-effective methods of natural healing. It is especially important today due to extensive exposure to toxic metals and chemicals.

Fifteen chapters cover sauna benefits, physiological effects, protocols, cautions, healing reactions, and many other aspects of sauna therapy.

Dr. Wilson is an instructor of Biochemistry, Hair Mineral Analysis, Sauna Therapy and Jurisprudence at various colleges and universities including Yamuni Institute of the Healing Arts (Maurice, LA), University of Natural Medicine (Santa Fe, NM), Natural Healers Academy (Morristown, NJ), and Westbrook University (West Virginia). His books are used as textbooks at East-West School of Herbology and Ohio College of Natural Health.

Paperback book, 8.5 x 11", 167 pages, $19.95

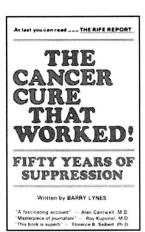

Book • $19.95

Over 50,000 Copies Sold!

The Cancer Cure That Worked: Fifty Years of Suppression

At Last You Can Read... The Rife Report

By Barry Lynes

Investigative journalism at its best. Barry Lynes takes readers on an exciting journey into the life work of Royal Rife. In 2008, we became the official distributor for this book. Call or visit us online for wholesale terms.

"A fascinating account..."
-Alan Cantwell, MD

"This book is superb."
-Florence B. Seibert, PhD

"Barry Lynes is one of the greatest health reporters in our country. With the assistance of John Crane, longtime friend and associate of Roy Rife, Barry has produced a masterpiece..." -Roy Kupsinel, M.D., editor of *Health Consciousness Journal*

Paperback book, 5 x 8", 169 pages, $19.95

Rife Video Documentary
2-Part DVD Set, Produced by
Zero Zero Two Productions

Must-Have DVD set for your Rife technology education!

In 1999, a stack of forgotten audio tapes was discovered. On the tapes were the voices of several people at the center of the events which are the subject of this documentary: a revolutionary treatment for cancer and a practical cure for all infectious disease.

The audio tapes were over 40 years old. The voices on them had almost faded, nearly losing key details of perhaps the most important medical story of the 20th Century.

But due to the efforts of the Kinnaman Foundation, the faded tapes have been restored and the voices on them recovered. So now, even though the participants have all passed away...

...they can finally tell their story.

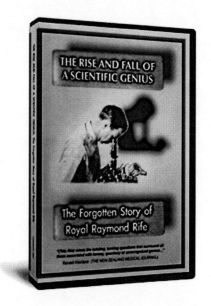

2-part DVD Set • $39.95

"These videos are great. We show them at the Annual Rife International Health Conference."
-Richard Loyd, Ph.D.

"A mind-shifting experience for those of us indoctrinated with a conventional view of biology."
-Townsend Letter for Doctors and Patients

In the summer of 1934 at a special medical clinic in La Jolla, California, sixteen patients withering from terminal disease were given a new lease on life. It was the first controlled application of a new electronic treatment for cancer: the Beam Ray Machine.

Within ninety days all sixteen patients walked away from the clinic, signed-off by the attending doctors as cured.

What followed the incredible success of this revolutionary treatment was not a welcoming by the scientific community, but a sad tale of its ultimate suppression.

The Rise and Fall of a Scientific Genius documents the scientific ignorance, official corruption, and personal greed directed at the inventor of the Beam Ray Machine, Royal Raymond Rife, forcing him and his inventions out of the spotlight and into obscurity. **Just converted from VHS to DVD and completely updated.**

Do not miss this opportunity to educate yourself about the history of rife technology!

Includes bonus DVD with interviews and historical photographs! Produced in Canada.

2 DVD-set, including bonus DVD, $39.95

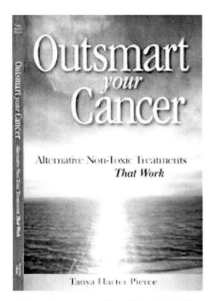

Book and Audio CD • $24.50

Outsmart Your Cancer: Alternative Non-Toxic Treatments That Work

By Tanya Harter Pierce

Note: Although Lymebook.com primarily focuses on books and resources for Lyme Disease, we know that cancer affects many of our customers. Consequently, we offer this excellent book/audio CD set on alternative cancer therapy.

Publisher's Remarks:

Why BLUDGEON cancer to death with common conventional treatments that can be toxic and harmful to your entire body?

When you OUTSMART your cancer, only the cancer cells die — NOT your healthy cells!

OUTSMART YOUR CANCER: Alternative Non-Toxic Treatments That Work is an easy guide to successful non-toxic treatments for cancer that you can obtain right now! In it, you will read real-life stories of people who have completely recovered from their advanced or late-stage lung cancer, breast cancer, prostate cancer, kidney cancer, brain cancer, childhood leukemia, and other types of cancer using effective non-toxic approaches.

This book explains the successful approaches these people used. It also gives you the resources to obtain these treatments right now, including a list of phone numbers and answers to questions about financial cost.

You will also learn other valuable information, such as:

"As a doctor practicing alternative medicine, I recommend this book to anyone that is involved with cancer."
- Dr. L. Durrett

- The unique characteristics of cancer cells that can be exploited to "outsmart" cancer.
- How to evaluate mainstream conventional treatments and what questions to ask your doctor.
- What women need to know about their hormones and cancer.
- How to alkalize your body and why this matters, both for prevention and treatment of cancer.
- Many of the causes of cancer that are increasingly common in our modern world.
- How and why many of the best alternative treatments for cancer have been suppressed.
- How to cope with the fear that comes with a cancer diagnosis.

Plus, *OUTSMART YOUR CANCER* is one of the few books in print today that gives a complete description of the amazing formula called "Protocel," which has produced incredible cancer recoveries over the past 20 years! A supporting audio CD is included with this book. Pricing = $19.95 book + $5.00 CD.

Paperback book, 6 x 9", 437 pages, with audio CD, $24.95

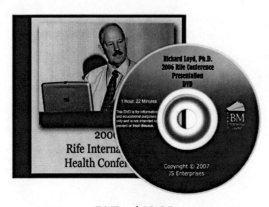

DVD • $19.95

Richard Loyd, Ph.D., presents at the Rife International Health Conference in Seattle

Watch this DVD to gain a better understanding of the technical details of rife technology.

Dr. Loyd, who earned a Ph.D. in nutrition, has researched and experimented with numerous electrotherapeutic devices, including the Rife/Bare unit, various EMEM machines, F-Scan, BioRay, magnetic pulsers, Doug Machine, and more. Dr. Loyd also has a wealth of knowledge in the use of herbs and supplements to support Rife electromagnetics.

By watching this DVD, you will discover the nuts and bolts of some very important, yet little known, principles of rife machine operation, including:

- Gating, sweeping, session time
- Square vs. sine wave
- DC vs. AC frequencies
- Duty cycle
- Octaves and scalar octaves

- Voltage variations and radio frequencies
- Explanation of the spark gap
- Contact vs. radiant mode
- Stainless vs. copper contacts
- A unique look at various frequency devices

DVD, 59 minutes, $19.95

The 2008 Lyme Disease Annual Report, by Bryan Rosner and Contributing Writers

This book serves as Bryan Rosner's annual newsletter.

The 2008 report covers numerous topics, including glyconutrient supplementation, updates on rife machine treatment planning and machine manufacturers, evidence supporting the existence of chronic Lyme Disease as a real medical condition, statistics indicating the presence of Lyme Disease on all

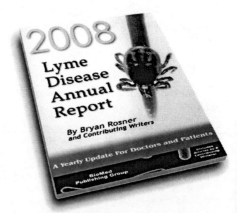

Paperback Book • $19.95

continents of the planet, and much more. Includes articles by 6 contributing writers: **James Schaller, M.D., Richard Brand, M.D., Sue Vogan, Ginger Savely, FNP-C, Tami Duncan, Susan Williams, and Richard Loyd, Ph.D.** Stay up to date!

Paperback book, 7 x 10", 168 pages, $19.95

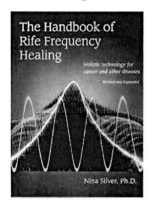

Book • $60

The Handbook of Rife Frequency Healing: Holistic Technology for Cancer and Other Diseases

By Nenah Sylver, PhD

This is the most complete, authoritative Rife technology handbook in the world. Weighing over 2 lbs., and 448 pages long, a broad range of topics are covered:

- Little-known differences between allopathic (Western) medicine and holistic health care
- Royal Raymond Rife's life, inventions, ideas and relationships
- Frequently Asked Questions about Rife sessions and equipment, with extensive session information
- Ground-breaking information on strengthening and supporting the body, based on years of research by the author
- A 200-page, cross-referenced Frequency Directory including hundreds of health conditions
- Bibliography, Three Appendices, Historical Photos, and MUCH MORE!

Paperback book, 8.5 x 11", 430 pages, $60

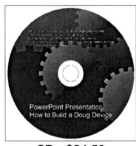

CD • $24.50

PowerPoint Presentation on CD
How to Build a Coil Machine

Of all rife machines used to fight Lyme Disease, the Coil Machine (also known as the Doug Device or QSC1850HD Device) has the longest and most established track record. This PowerPoint presentation was put together by the husband of a Lyme Disease sufferer who built the machine for his wife. It provides construction information, parts sourcing, and a detailed schematic. Now you can build your own Coil Machine!

Microsoft PowerPoint Presentation on CD, $24.50

Ordering Options
- **Toll Free (866) 476-7637**
- **www.LymeBookStore.com**

Call today to place an order or request additional catalogs. Detailed product information and secure online ordering is available on our website.

Do you have a book inside you? We are looking for new authors of books on Lyme Disease, alternative medicine, and related topics. Find out more and submit your book proposal online at www.LymeBook.com/submit-book-proposal.

Join Lyme Community Forums (www.lymecommunity.com), a new online discussion group, to communicate for FREE with fellow Lyme sufferers!

DISCLAIMER: Our products are for informational and educational purposes only. They are not intended to prevent, diagnose, treat, or cure disease.

INDEX

of Psychological Medicine   78, 120

K

Kazuko Curtin   54-7, 66
Kidneys   63, 238
Kindergarten   20, 22
Kinesiology   214
Klebs, Edwin   36
Klimas, Nancy   52
Klinghardt, Dietrich, M.D., Ph.D.   14, 24
Knees   35-6, 63, 233
Krebs cycle issues   174
Kucera, John   198-9

L

Lab work   168, 173, 201-2, 217
Lancet   vi, 121
Language, development   40, 105, 211-2, 223
Larsson, Christer   vii
Laser treatment   215, 227
Law, Paul A.   75
Learning deficits   241
Leptospirosis   71, 108
Lesions   63, 92, 200
Levin, Warren   14, 106, 198
L-form bacteria   168
LIAF (Lyme Induced Autism Foundation)   iv, ix, 11, 13-6, 18, 25-6, 28, 44, 61, 75, 104, 106, 151-3, 159, 197-9, 205
Liver   24, 63-4, 190, 238-9
LLMDs (Lyme-Literate Medical Doctor)   x, 24, 50, 152-4, 156, 158, 160, 183-4, 198, 221, 233-5
Load
  bacterial   99
  viral   173
Love, Janelle   14
Luepker, Ian R.   14
Lump   245
Lungs   87, 89
Lupus   221
Lupus   76
Lyme disease, acute   48, 72
Lyme Disease Annual Report   70, 162
Lyme Disease Association   160
Lyme Disease Association Doctor Referral Service   156
Lyme Disease Solution, Book by Kenneth Singleton, M.D.   162
Lyme titer   170
Lymenet.org   156
Lymphocyte blastogenesis assay   87

W

X

Y

Z

Don't Miss BioMed Publishing Group's
Newest Lyme Disease Books!

*The Lyme Disease Survival Guide:
Physical, Lifestyle, and Emotional Strategies
for Healing*

By Connie Strasheim

*The Experts of Lyme Disease:
A Radio Journalist Visits the Front Lines of
The Lyme Wars*

By Sue Vogan

Available from www.LymeBook.com

CPSIA information can be obtained at www.ICGtesting.com
Printed in the USA
BVOW03s1849141113

336249BV00001B/42/P